Food Poisoning

Edwin Oakes Jordan

CONTENTS

CHAPTER PAGE

Rachitis The Foods Most Commonly Poisonous

CHAPTER I

INTRODUCTION

How frequently food poisoning occurs is not definitely known. Everybody is aware that certain articles of food are now and again held responsible for more or less severe "attacks of indigestion" or other physiological disturbances that have followed their consumption, but in many cases the evidence for assuming a causal connection is of the slightest. That convenient refuge from etiological uncertainty, "ptomain poisoning," is a diagnosis that unquestionably has been made to cover a great variety of diverse conditions, from appendicitis and the pain caused by gallstones to the simple abdominal distention resulting from reckless gorging.

No doubt can be entertained, however, that intestinal and other disorders due to particular articles of food occur much more frequently than they are recorded. There are few persons who have not experienced gastro-intestinal attacks of moderate severity which could be reasonably attributed to something eaten shortly before. It is often possible to specify with a fair degree of certainty the offending food. The great majority of such attacks are of a mild character, are quickly recovered from, and are never heard of beyond the immediate family circle. Only when the attack is more serious than the average or when a large number of persons are affected simultaneously does knowledge of the occurrence become more widely spread. A small proportion of food-poisoning cases receives notice in the public press and a still smaller proportion is reported in the medical journals. Very few indeed are ever completely investigated as to their origin.

Although most attacks of food poisoning are usually of a slight and apparently temporary nature, it does not follow that they are to be considered negligible or of trivial importance from the standpoint of public health. The human organism is always more or less weakened by such attacks, many of them, as we shall see, genuine infections; and, as is known to be the case with many infectious diseases, some permanent injurious impression may be left on the body of the affected individual. Under certain conditions it is possible that degenerative changes are initiated or accelerated in the kidneys or blood vessels by the acute poisoning which is manifested for a short time in even the milder cases. In yet greater degree these changes may follow those insidious forms of food poisoning due to the frequent ingestion of small quantities of mineral or organic poisons, which in each dose may cause little or no measurable physiological change, but whose cumulative effect may be vicious. In view of the grave situation evidenced by the increase in the degenerative diseases affecting early middle life in the United States,[1] the extent, causes, and means of prevention of food poisoning seem pressing subjects for investigation.

THE EXTENT OF FOOD POISONING

Since cases of food poisoning, "ptomain poisoning," and the like are not required by law to be reported, public health authorities in general possess no information respecting their occurrence. Very indirect and imperfect indications of the prevalence of certain kinds of food poisoning are afforded by casual press reports. Such as they are, these accounts are the only available material. Tables I and II summarize data I have gathered through a press-clipping bureau and other sources during the period October, 1913, to October, 1915. They serve to show at least the universality and complexity of the problem.

The 375 group and family outbreaks together involved 5,238 persons. While it is not probable that all the instances reported as due to food poisoning can properly be so considered, there is no doubt that the number recorded in the tables falls far short of the actual occurrences. In the past few years the writer has investigated several large food-poisoning outbreaks which have never been reported in the press nor received public notice in any way. There is reason to think that the majority of cases escape notice. Probably several thousand outbreaks of food poisoning in families and larger groups, affecting at least 15,000-20,000 persons, occur in the United States in the course of a year.

The assignment of causes indicated in Table I is of limited value. The tendency to incriminate canned food is here manifest. Proper investigation of the origin of an outbreak is so rarely carried out that the articles of food ordinarily accused are selected rather as the result of popular prejudice and tradition than of any careful inquiry.

TABLE I

FOOD POISONING IN THE UNITED STATES, OCTOBER, 1913, TO OCTOBER, 1915

Assigned cause	Group and Family	Individual	Total	Outbreaks	Cases	Total
Meat	40	35	75			
Canned fish	29	35	64			
Canned vegetables	27	34	61			
Ice cream	31	22	53			
Fish, oysters	17	31	48			
Cheese	31	9	40			
Sausage and canned meat	18	18	36			
Milk	14	13	27			
Mushrooms	12	7	19			
Fruit	8	11	19			
Vegetables	11	7	18			
Fowl	12	4	16			
Salad	9	5	14			
Contact of food or drink with metal	12	1	13			
Miscellaneous	29	55	84			
	300	287	587			
No cause assigned	357	88	445	657	375	1,032

TABLE II

SEASONAL DISTRIBUTION OF FOOD POISONING CASES, 1914-15 (GROUP, FAMILY, AND INDIVIDUAL)

January	90		May	63		September	76
February	66		June	108		October	96
March	75		July	99		November	96
April	79		August	96		December	88

There is no very striking seasonal incidence apparent in the figures here gathered (Table II). The warmer months seem to have a slight preponderance of cases, but general conclusions from such data are hardly warranted.

VARIOUS KINDS OF FOOD POISONING

Cases of poisoning by articles of food may be distinguished as: (1) those caused by some injurious constituent in the food itself, and (2) those caused by a peculiar condition of the individual consuming the food, by virtue of which essentially wholesome food substances are capable of producing physiological disturbance in certain individuals. The latter group includes persons, apparently normal in other respects, who are more or less injuriously affected by some particular article of diet, such as eggs or milk, which is eaten with impunity by all normal individuals. This is the so-called food sensitization or food allergy.

Food poisoning, as more commonly understood, is due to the composition, contents, or contamination of the food itself. It is not within the scope of this book to consider any of those cases in which definite poisonous substances are added to food with criminal intent. The term food poisoning is here taken to include the occasional cases of poisoning from organic poisons present in normal animal or plant tissues, the more or less injurious consequences following the consumption of food into which formed mineral or organic poisons have been introduced by accident or with intent to improve appearances or keeping quality, the cases of infection due to the swallowing of bacteria and other parasites which infest or contaminate certain foods, and the poisoning due to deleterious substances produced in food by the growth of bacteria, molds, and similar organisms. As already pointed out, little is known about the relative frequency of occurrence of these different causes or the extent to which they are separately and collectively operative.

THE ARTICLES OF FOOD MOST COMMONLY CONNECTED WITH FOOD POISONING

In addition to the definitely poisonous plants or animals, certain everyday articles of food have been frequently associated with the more serious outbreaks of food poisoning. Meat in particular has been implicated so often that the term meat poisoning is used about as commonly as the term food poisoning in general discussions of this subject. Certain it is that the great majority of the best-studied and most severe outbreaks of food poisoning have been attributed on good grounds to the use of meat or meat products. Other animal foods, and especially milk and its derivatives, cheese and ice-cream, have likewise been held responsible for extensive and notable outbreaks.

Perhaps the most significant feature of food poisoning attacks is the frequency with which they have been traced to the use of raw or imperfectly cooked food. The probable interpretation of this fact will be discussed in the later chapters. Especially have the use of uncooked milk, either by itself or mixed with other food substances, and the eating of raw sausage brought in their train symptoms of poisoning in a disproportionately large number of cases.

Canned goods of various sorts have likewise been repeatedly accused of causing injurious effects, but the evidence adduced is not always convincing. The actual degree of danger from this source is far from being determined. The National Canners Association publishes in the annual report of the secretary a brief list of "libels on the industry" or instances in which canned foods of various sorts were regarded as the cause of illness. The 1916 report contains fifty-one cases of this character, none of which was considered by the investigator of the Association to be based on sound evidence. A still more searching investigation of all such cases would seem to be desirable, not with a view to incriminating or exculpating any particular product, but simply for the purpose of ascertaining and placing on record all the facts.

FOOTNOTES:

[1] Tables A and B show that the "expectation of life" for adults of forty years and over is shorter in New York City now than it was thirty years ago (Table A), and that this increase in the death-rate in the higher-age groups is manifested in recent years in a wide area in this country (Table B). This increased mortality is due chiefly to diseases of the heart, arteries, and kidneys, and to cancer.

TABLE A[1a]

APPROXIMATE LIFE TABLE, TRIENNA 1879-81 AND 1909-11, BASED ON NEW YORK CITY STATISTICS

```
=======================================================
|Expectation|Expectation| Gain (+) or | of Life, | of Life, |Loss (-) in Years
Ages | 1879-81 | 1909-11 | of Expectancy --------+-----------+-----------+-----------
----- Under 5 | 41.3 | 51.9 | +10.6 5 | 46.3 | 51.1 | + 4.8 10 | 43.8 | 46.9 | +
3.1 15 | 39.7 | 42.5 | + 2.8 20 | 35.8 | 38.3 | + 2.5 25 | 32.6 | 34.3 | + 1.7 30
| 29.6 | 30.5 | + 0.9 35 | 26.7 | 26.9 | + 0.2 40 | 23.0 | 23.4 | - 0.5 45 | 21.1 |
20.0 | - 1.1 50 | 18.3 | 16.8 | - 1.5 55 | 15.4 | 13.9 | - 1.5 60 | 13.0 | 11.3 | -
1.7 65 | 10.5 | 9.1 | - 1.4 70 | 8.9 | 7.2 | - 1.7 75 | 7.3 | 5.5 | - 1.8 80 | 6.4 |
4.3 | - 2.1 85 | 5.5 | 2.2 | - 3.3 Balance | | | +26.6 | | | -16.6 | | |----------------
- | | | +10.0 --------------------------------------------------
```

TABLE B[1b]

COMPARISON OF MORTALITY OF MALES AND FEMALES, BY AGE GROUPS. DEATH-RATES PER 1,000 POPULATION (REGISTRATION STATES AS CONSTITUTED IN 1900)

```
================================================================
Ages | Males |Percentage | Females |Percentage |-----------|Increase or|------
-----|Increase or | 1900| 1911| Decrease | 1900| 1911| Decrease -------------+-
----+-----+-----------+----------------------- Under 5 | 54.2| 39.8| -26.27 | 45.8|
33.3| -27.29 5-9 | 4.7| 3.4| -27.66 | 4.6| 3.1| -32.61 10-14 | 2.9| 2.4| -17.24
```

| 3.1| 2.1| -32.26 15-19 | 4.9| 3.7| -24.49 | 4.8| 3.3| -31.25 20-24 | 7.0| 5.3| -24.29 | 6.7| 4.7| -29.85 25-34 | 8.3| 6.7| -19.28 | 8.2| 6.0| -26.83 35-44 | 10.8| 10.4| -3.70 | 9.8| 8.3| -15.31 45-54 | 15.8| 16.1| +1.90 | 14.2| 12.9| -9.15 55-64 | 28.9| 30.9| +6.92 | 25.8| 26.8| +0.78 65-74 | 59.6| 61.6| +3.36 | 53.8| 55.1| +2.42 75 and over|146.1|147.4| +0.89 |139.5|139.2| +0.22 All ages | 17.6| 15.8| -10.23 | 16.5| 14.0| -15.15 ---------------------------- --------------------------------

[1a] Monthly Bull., Dept. of Health, City of New York, III (1913), 113.

[1b] Dublin, Amer. Jour. Public Health, III (1915), 1262.

CHAPTER II

SENSITIZATION TO PROTEIN FOODS

The first introduction under the skin of a guinea-pig of a minute quantity of egg-white or other apparently harmless protein substance is itself without visible injurious effect, but if this is followed by a second injection of the same substance after an interval of about ten days, the animal will die in a few minutes with symptoms of violent poisoning. Whatever be the physiological explanation of the remarkable change that thus results from the incorporation of foreign protein into the body, there can be no doubt that the phenomenon known as protein sensitization or anaphylaxis is relatively common.[2] Sensitization to proteins came to light in the first instance through the study of therapeutic sera, and has been found to have unexpectedly wide bearings. It is now known that not only the rash and other symptoms which sometimes follow the administration of horse serum containing diphtheria antitoxin, but the reaction to tuberculin and similar accompaniments of bacterial infection, are probably to be explained on the principle of anaphylactic change. The sensitiveness of certain individuals to the pollen of particular plants (hay fever) is also regarded as a typical instance of anaphylaxis, accompanied as it is by asthma and other characteristic manifestations of the anaphylactic condition.

Among the reactions usually classed as anaphylactic are the occasional cases of sensitivity to particular food substances. It is a familiar fact that certain foods that can be eaten with impunity by most persons prove more or less acutely poisonous for others. Strawberries and some other fruits and some kinds of shellfish are among the articles of food more commonly implicated. Unpleasant reactions to the use of eggs and of cow's milk are also noted. The severity of the attacks may vary from a slight rash to violent gastro-intestinal, circulatory, and nervous disturbances.

Coues[3] has described a rather typical case in a child twenty-one months old and apparently healthy except for some eczema. When the child was slightly over a year old egg-white was given to it, and nausea and vomiting immediately followed. About eight months later another feeding with egg-white was followed by sneezing and all the symptoms of an acute coryza. Extensive urticaria covering most of the body also appeared, and the eyelids became edematous. The temperature remained normal and there was no marked prostration. The symptoms of such attacks vary considerably in different individuals, but usually include pronounced urticaria along with nausea, vomiting, and diarrhea. The rapidity with which the symptoms appear after eating is highly characteristic. Schloss[4] has reported a case of an eight-year-old boy who evinced marked sensitiveness to eggs, almonds, and oatmeal. Experiments in this instance showed that a reaction was produced only by the proteins of these several foods, and that extracts and preparations free from protein were entirely inert. It was further found that by injection of the patient's blood serum guinea-pigs could be passively sensitized against the substances in question, thus showing the condition to be one of real anaphylaxis.

Idiosyncrasy to cow's milk which is observed sometimes in infants is an anaphylactic phenomenon.[5] The substitution of goat's milk for cow's milk has been followed by favorable results in such cases.

In very troublesome cases of protein idiosyncrasy a method of treatment based on animal experimentation has been advocated. This consists in the production of a condition of "anti-anaphylaxis" by systematic feeding of minute doses of the specific protein substance concerned.[6] S. R. Miller[7] describes the case of a child in whom a constitutional reaction followed the administration of one teaspoonful of a mixture composed of one pint of water plus one drop of egg-white, while a like amount of albumen diluted with one quart of water was tolerated perfectly. "Commencing with the dilution which failed to produce a reaction, the child was given gradually increasing amounts of solutions of increasing strength. The dosage was always one teaspoonful given three times during the day; the result has been that, in a period of about three months, the child has been desensitized to such an extent that one dram of pure egg-white is now taken with impunity."

Many other instances of anaphylaxis to egg albumen are on record.[8] In some of these cases the amount of the specific protein that suffices to produce the reaction is exceedingly small. One physician writes of a patient who "was unable to take the smallest amount of egg in any form. If a spoon was used to beat eggs and then to stir his coffee, he became very much nauseated and vomited violently."[9]

The dependence of many cases of "asthma" upon particular foods is an established fact. Various skin rashes and eruptions are likewise associated with sensitization to certain foods.[10] McBride and Schorer[11] consider that each particular kind of food (as tomatoes or cereals) produces a constant and characteristic set of symptoms. Possibly certain definitely characterized skin diseases are due to this form of food poisoning. Blacktan[12] found that of forty-three patients without eczema only one showed any evidence of susceptibility to protein by cutaneous and intracutaneous tests, while of twenty-seven patients with eczema twenty-two gave evidence of susceptibility to proteins.

FOOTNOTES:

[2] General agreement respecting the true physiological and chemical

nature of anaphylactic phenomena has not yet been reached. For a discussion of the theories of anaphylaxis, see in Hans Zinsser, Infection and Resistance (New York, 1914), chaps. xv-xviii; also Doerr, "Allergie und Anaphylaxis," in Kolle and Wassermann, Handbuch, 2d edition, 1913, II, 947.

[3] Boston Med. and Surg. Jour., CLXVII (1912), 216.

[4] Amer. Jour. Obstet. (New York), LXV (1912), 731.

[5] F. B. Talbot, Boston Med. and Surg. Jour., CLXXV (1916), 409.

[6] See, for example, Schloss, loc. cit.

[7] Johns Hopkins Hosp. Bull., XXV (1914), 78.

[8] See, for example, K. Koessler, Ill. Med. Jour., XXIII (1913), 66; Bronfenbrenner, Andrews, and Scott, Jour. Amer. Med. Assoc., LXIV (1915), 1306; F. B. Talbot, Boston Med. and Surg. Jour., CLXXI (1914), 708.

[9] Jour. Amer. Med. Assoc., LXV (1915), 1837.

[10] Strickler and Goldberg, Jour. Amer. Med. Assoc., LXVI (1916), 249.

[11] Jour. Cutaneous Dis., XXXIV (1916), 70.

[12] Amer. Jour. Dis. of Children, XI (1916), 441.

CHAPTER III

POISONOUS PLANTS AND ANIMALS

Some normal plant and animal tissues contain substances poisonous to man and are occasionally eaten by mistake for wholesome foods.

POISONOUS PLANTS

Poisonous plants have sometimes figured conspicuously in human affairs. Every reader of ancient history knows how Socrates "drank the hemlock," and how crafty imperial murderers were likely to substitute poisonous mushrooms for edible ones in the dishes prepared for guests who were out of favor. In our own times the eating of poisonous plants is generally an accident, and poisoning from this cause occurs chiefly among the young and the ignorant.

According to Chesnut[13] there are 16,673 leaf-bearing plants included in Heller's Catalogue of North American Plants, and of these nearly five hundred, in one way or another, have been alleged to be poisonous. Some of these are relatively rare or for other reasons are not likely to be eaten by man or beast; others contain a poison only in some particular part, or are poisonous only at certain seasons of the year; in some the poison is not dangerous when taken by the mouth, but only when brought in contact with the skin or injected beneath the skin or into the circulation. There are great differences in individual susceptibility to some of these plant poisons. One familiar plant, the so-called poison-ivy, is not harmful for many people even when handled recklessly; it can be eaten with impunity by most domestic animals.

The actual number of poisonous plants likely to be inadvertently eaten by human beings is not large. Chesnut[14] has enumerated about thirty important poisonous plants occurring in the United States, and some of these are not known to be poisonous except for domestic animals.[15] Many of the cases of reported poisoning in man belong to the class of exceedingly rare accidents and are without much significance in the present discussion. Such are the use of the leaves of the American false hellebore (Veratrum viride) in mistake for those of the marsh-marigold[16], the use of the fruit pulp of the Kentucky coffee tree (Gymnocladus dioica) in mistake for that of the honey-locust[17], the accidental employment of daffodil bulbs for food, and the confusion by children of the young shoots of the broad-leaf laurel (Kalmia latifolia) with the wintergreen.[18] One of the most serious instances of poisoning of this sort is that from the use of the spindle-shaped roots of the deadly water hemlock (Cicuta maculata) allied to the more famous but no more deadly poison hemlock. These underground portions of the plant are sometimes exposed to view by washing out or freezing, and are mistaken by children for horseradish, artichokes, parsnips, and other edible roots. Poisoning with water hemlock undoubtedly occurs more frequently than shown by any record. Eight cases and two deaths from this cause are known to have occurred in one year in the state of New Jersey alone.

An instance of food poisoning to be included under this head is the outbreak in Hamburg and some thirty other German cities in 1911 due to the use of a poisonous vegetable fat in preparing a commercial butter substitute.[19] In the attempt to cheapen as far as possible the preparation of margarin various plant oils have been added by the manufacturers. In the Hamburg outbreak, in which over two hundred cases of illness occurred, poisoning was apparently due to substitution of so-called maratti-oil, derived from a tropical plant (Hydrocarpus). This fat is said to be identical with oil of cardamom, and its toxic character in the amounts used in the margarin was proved by animal experiment. Increasing economic pressure for cheap foods may lead to the recurrence of such accidents unless proper precautions are used in testing out new fats and other untried substances intended for use in the preparation of food substances.[20]

Investigators from the New York City Health Department have found that certain cases of alleged "ptomain poisoning" were really due to "sour-grass soup."[21] This soup is prepared from the leaves of a species of sorrel rich in oxalic acid. In one restaurant it was found that the soup contained as much as ten grains of oxalic acid per pint!

By far the best-known example of that form of poisoning which results from confounding poisonous with edible foods is that due to poisonous mushrooms.[22] There is reason to believe that mushroom (or "toadstool") intoxication in the United States has occurred with greater frequency of late years, partly on account of the generally increasing use of mushrooms as food and the consequently greater liability to mistake, and partly on account of the growth of immigration from the mushroom-eating communities of Southern Europe. Many instances have come to light in which immigrants have mistaken poisonous varieties in this country for edible ones with which they were familiar at home. In the vicinity of New York City there were twenty-two deaths from mushroom poisoning in one ten-day period (September, 1911) following heavy rains. The "fly Amanita"[23] (Amanita muscaria) in this country has been apparently often mistaken for the European variety of "royal Amanita" (A. caesaria).[24] Such a mistake seems to have been the cause of death of the Count de Vecchi in Washington, D.C., in 1897.

The Count, an attache of the Italian legation, a cultivated gentleman of nearly sixty years of age, considered something of an expert upon mycology, purchased, near one of the markets in Washington, a quantity of fungi recognized by him as an edible mushroom. The plants were collected in Virginia about seven miles from the city of Washington. The following Sunday morning the count and his physician, a warm personal friend, breakfasted together upon these mushrooms, commenting upon their agreeable and even delicious flavor. Breakfast was concluded at half after eight and within fifteen minutes the count felt symptoms of serious illness. So rapid was the onset that by nine o'clock he was found prostrate on his bed, oppressed by the sense of impending doom. He rapidly developed blindness, trismus, difficulty in swallowing, and shortly lost consciousness. Terrific convulsions then supervened, so violent in character as to break the bed upon which he was placed. Despite rigorous treatment and the administration of morphine and atropine, the count never recovered consciousness and died on the day following the accident. The count's physician on returning to his office was also attacked, dizziness and ocular symptoms warning him of the nature of the trouble. Energetic treatment with apomorphine and atropine was at once instituted by his colleagues and for a period of five hours he lay in a state of coma with occasional periods of lucidity. The grave symptoms were ameliorated and recovery set in somewhere near seven o'clock in the evening. His convalescence was uneventful, his restoration to health complete, and he is, I believe, still living. On this instance the count probably identified the fungi as caesaria or aurantiaca. From the symptoms and termination the species eaten must have been muscaria.

A. muscaria contains an alkaloidal substance which has a characteristic effect upon the nerve centers and to which the name muscarin and the provisional chemical formula $C_5H_{15}NO_3$ has been given. The drug atropin is a more or less perfect physiological antidote for muscarin and has been administered with success in cases of muscarin poisoning. It is said that the peasants in the Caucasus are in the habit of preparing from the fly Amanita a beverage which they use for producing orgies of intoxication. Deaths are stated to occur frequently from excessive use of this beverage.[25]

The deadly Amanita or death-cup (A. phalloides) is probably responsible for the majority of cases of mushroom poisoning. Ford estimates that from twelve to fifteen deaths occur annually in this country from this species alone. This fungus is usually eaten through sheer ignorance by persons who have gathered and eaten whatever they chanced to find in the woods. A few of these poisonous mushrooms mixed with edible varieties may be sufficient to cause the death of a family. Ford thus describes the symptoms of poisoning with A. phalloides:

Following the consumption of the fungi there is a period of six to fifteen hours during which no symptoms of poisoning are shown by the victims. This corresponds to the period of incubation of other intoxications or infections. The first sign of trouble is sudden pain of the greatest intensity localized in the abdomen, accompanied by vomiting, thirst, and choleraic diarrhoea with mucous and bloody stools. The latter symptom is by no means constant. The pain continues in paroxysms often so severe as to cause the peculiar Hippocratic facies, la face vultueuse of the French, and though sometimes ameliorated in character, it usually recurs with greater severity. The patients rapidly lose strength and flesh, their complexion assuming a peculiar yellow tone. After three to four days in children and six to eight in adults the victims sink into a profound coma from which they cannot be roused and death soon ends the fearful and useless tragedy. Convulsions rarely if ever occur and when present indicate, I am inclined to believe, a mixed intoxication, specimens of Amanita muscaria being eaten with the phalloides. The majority of individuals poisoned by the "deadly Amanita" die, the mortality varying from 60 to 100 per cent in various accidents, but recovery is not impossible when small amounts of the fungus are eaten, especially if the stomach be very promptly emptied, either naturally or artificially.

A number of other closely related species of Amanita (e.g., A. verna, the "destroying angel," probably a small form of A. phalloides) have a poisonous action similar to that of A. phalloides. All are different from muscarin.

The character of the poison was first carefully investigated by Kobert, who showed that the Amanita extract has the power of laking or dissolving out the coloring matter from red blood corpuscles. This hemolytic action is so powerful that it is exerted upon the red cells of ox blood even in a dilution of 1:125,000. Ford[26] has since shown that in addition to the hemolytic substance another substance much more toxic is present in this species of Amanita and he concludes that the poisonous effect of the fungus is primarily due to the latter ("Amanita toxin"). The juice of the cooked Amanita is devoid of hemolytic power, but is poisonous for animals in small doses, a fact that agrees with the observation that these mushrooms, after cooking, remain intensely poisonous for man. Extensive fatty degeneration in liver, kidney, and heart muscle is produced by the true Amanita toxin. In the Baltimore cases studied by Clark, Marshall, and Rowntree[27] the kidney rather than the liver was the seat of the most interesting functional changes. These authors conclude that the nervous and mental symptoms, instead of being due to some peculiar "neurotoxin," are probably uremic in character. No successful method of treatment is known. An antibody for the hemolysin has been produced, but an antitoxin for the other poisonous substance seems to be formed in very small amount. Attempts to immunize small animals with Amanita toxin succeed only to a limited degree.[28]

POISONOUS ANIMALS

While the muscles or internal organs of many animals are not palatable on account of unpleasant flavor or toughness, there do not seem to be many instances in which normal animal tissues are poisonous when eaten. As pointed out elsewhere (chapter vi), the majority of outbreaks of meat and fish poisoning must be attributed to the presence of pathogenic bacteria or to poisons formed after the death of the animal. This has been found especially true of many of the outbreaks of poisoning ascribed to oysters and other shellfish; in most, if not all, cases the inculpated mollusks have been derived from water polluted with human wastes and are either infected or partially decomposed.

In some animals, however, notably certain fish, the living and healthy organs are definitely poisonous. The family of Tetrodontidae (puffers, balloon-fish, globe-fish) comprises a number of poisonous species, including the famous Japanese Fugu, which has many hundred deaths scored against it and has been often used to effect suicide. Poisonous varieties of fish seem more abundant in tropical waters than in temperate, but this is possibly because of the more general and indiscriminate use of fish as food in such localities as the Japanese and South Sea Islands. It is known that some cool-water fish are poisonous. The flesh of the Greenland shark possesses poisonous qualities for dogs and produces a kind of intoxication in these animals.[29]

Much uncertainty exists respecting the conditions under which the various forms of fish poisoning occur. One type is believed to be associated with the spawning season, and to be caused by a poison present in the reproductive tissues. The roe of the European barbel is said to cause frequent poisoning, not usually of a serious sort. The flesh or roe of the sturgeon, pike, and other fish is also stated to be poisonous during the spawning season. Some fish are said to be poisonous only when they have fed on certain marine plants.[30]

There is little definite knowledge about the poisons concerned. They are certainly not uniform in nature. The Fugu poison produces cholera-like symptoms, convulsions, and paralysis. It is not destroyed by boiling. The effect of the Greenland shark flesh on dogs is described as being "like alcohol." It is said that dogs fed with gradually increasing amounts of the poisonous shark's flesh become to some degree immune. Different symptoms are described in other fish poisoning cases.[31]

FOOTNOTES:

[13] Science, XV (1902), 1016.

[14] U.S. Dept. of Agric., Div. of Botany, Bull. 20, 1898.

[15] Among the plants that seem to be most commonly implicated in the poisoning of stock are the larkspur (Delphinium. U.S. Dept. of Agric., Bull. 365, September 8, 1916), the water hemlock (Cicuta maculata) and others of the same genus, the lupines (U.S. Dept. of Agric., Bull. 405, 1916), some of the laurels (Kalmia), and the Death Camas or Zygadenus (U.S. Dept. of Agric., Bull. 125, 1915). The famous loco-weed of the western United States (U.S. Dept. of Agric., Bull. 112, 1909) is less certainly to be held responsible for all the ills ascribed to it (H. T. Marshall, Johns Hopkins Hosp. Bull., XXV [1914], 234).

[16] Chesnut, U.S. Dept. of Agric., Div. of Botany, Bull. 20, 1898, p. 17.

[17] Ibid., p. 28.

[18] Ibid., p. 45. The seeds of the castor-oil bean, which contain a very powerful poison (ricin) allied to the bacterial toxins, have been known to cause the death of children who ate the seeds given them to play with.

[19] Mayer, Deutsche Viertelj. fentl. Ges., XLV (1913), 12.

[20] Cf. an instance of palmolin poisoning, Centralbl. f. Bakt., I, Ref., LXII (1914), 210.

[21] Weekly Bull., N.Y. Dept. of Health, September 16, 1916.

[22] Seventy-three species of mushrooms known or suspected to be poisonous are enumerated in a bulletin of the United States Department of Agriculture, Patterson and Charles ("Mushrooms and Other Common Fungi," Bull. 175, 1915). This bulletin contains descriptions and excellent illustrations of many edible and of the commoner poisonous species.

[23] Used in some places as a fly poison.

[24] Ford, Science, XXX (1909), 97.

[25] Another species of mushroom occurring in this country and commonly regarded as edible (Panaeolus papilionaceus) has on occasion shown marked intoxicating properties (A. E. Verrill, Science, XL (1914), 408).

[26] Jour. Infect. Dis., III (1906), 191.

[27] Jour. Amer. Med. Assoc., LXIV (1915), 1230.

[28] W. W. Ford, "Plant Poisons and Their Antibodies," Centralbl. f. Bakt., I Abt., Ref., LVIII (1913), 129 and 193, with full bibliography.

[29] A. H. Clark, Science, XLI (1915), 795.

[30] See W. M. Kerr, U.S. Nav., Monthly Bull., VI (1912), 401.

[31] Ibid.

CHAPTER IV

MINERAL OR ORGANIC POISONS ADDED TO FOOD

Well-known mineral or organic poisons--"chemical poisons"--sometimes find their way into food, being either introduced accidentally in the process of manufacture or preparation, or being added deliberately with intent to improve the appearance or keeping qualities of the food.

ARSENIC

So powerful a poison as arsenic has been occasionally introduced into food by stupidity or carelessness. Arsenic has been found by English authorities to be generally present in food materials dried or roasted with gases arising from the combustion of coal, and in materials treated with sulphuric acid during the process of preparation. In both cases the source is the same: the iron pyrites, practically always arsenical, contained in the coal or used in making the sulphuric acid.

A celebrated epidemic of "peripheral neuritis" in the English Midlands in 1900 was traced to the presence of dangerous quantities of arsenic in beer. About six thousand persons were affected in this outbreak and there were some seventy deaths. The beer coming from the suspected breweries had all been manufactured with the use of brewing sugars obtained from a single source, and these sugars were found to have been impregnated with arsenic by the sulphuric acid used in their preparation, some specimens of the acid containing as much as 2.6 per cent of arsenic.[32]

The use of glucose, not only in beer, but as an admixture or adulterant in jams, syrups, candies, and the like, is open to serious objection unless the glucose is known to have been prepared with sulphuric acid freed from arsenical impurity. In fact, the use of any food material prepared by the aid of sulphuric acid is permissible only in case arsenic-free acid is employed.[33]

ANTIMONY

The cheaper grades of enameled cooking utensils in use in this country contain antimony, and this is dissolved out in noteworthy amounts in cooking various foods.[34] The rubber nipples used for infants' milk bottles also sometimes contain antimony.[35] Although the poisonous qualities of antimony are well known, there is little information about the toxic effect of repeated very minute doses. Recognized instances of chronic antimony poisoning are very rare. Further investigation is needed.

LEAD

The well-known poisonousness of lead and its compounds prevents, as a rule, the deliberate addition of lead salts to food substances, although it is true that lead chromate is sometimes used for imparting a yellow color to candy and decorating sugars.[36] Foods that are wrapped in foil, however, such as chocolate and soft cheese, contain traces of lead, as do the contents of preserve jars with metallic caps and the "soft drinks" vended in bottles with patent metal stoppers. Occasional ingestion of minute quantities of lead is probably a matter of little physiological importance, but since lead is a cumulative poison, frequent taking into the body of even very small amounts entails danger. Severe lead poisoning has been known to result from the habitual use of acid beverages contained in bottles with lead stoppers. Investigations made to determine the possible danger of poisoning from lead taken up from glazed and earthenware cooking utensils indicate that injury from this source is unlikely. The enameled ware in common use in this country is lead-free.

Objection on the ground of possible contamination has been raised to the use of solder for sealing food cans. Such objections have less weight than formerly owing to changes in the construction of the container, so that any contact of solder with the food is now minimized and to a large extent done away with altogether.

In consequence of the fact that many natural waters attack lead, the use of lead service pipes for wells, cisterns, and public water supplies has given rise to numerous outbreaks of lead poisoning. It is now generally recognized that water intended for drinking purposes should not be drawn through lead pipes.

A special liability to take lead into the stomach exists in persons working at the painters' trade and other occupations involving contact with lead and its salts. It has been shown that the eating of food handled with paint-smeared hands brings about the ingestion of considerable quantities of lead and, when long continued, results in lead poisoning. The risk of contaminating food with lead in this way can be greatly lessened by thorough cleansing of the hands with soap and hot water before eating.[37]

TIN

Special interest has attached to the possibility of tin poisoning on account of the widespread use of canned foods.[38] It is established chemically that tin is attacked, not only by acid fruits and berries, but by some vegetables having only a slightly acid reaction. More tin is found in the drained solids than in the liquor, and the metal is largely in an insoluble form.[39] It has been the general opinion based on experiments by Lehmann[40] and others that the amounts of tin ordinarily present in canned foods "are undeserving of serious notice," and this view has found expression in the leading textbooks on hygiene.[41] Certainly there has not been any noticeable amount of tin poisoning observed coincident with the enormous increase in the use of canned foods. An instance of poisoning by canned asparagus observed by Friedmann,[42] however, is attributed by him to the tin content, and this view is rendered probable by the negative result of his bacteriological and serological examinations. Canned asparagus apparently contains an unusually large amount of soluble tin compounds.[43] There seems some ground for the assumption that certain individuals are especially susceptible to small quantities of tin and that the relative infrequency of such cases as that cited by Friedmann can be best explained in this way. Lacquered or "enamel lined" cans are being used to an increasing extent for fruits and vegetables that are especially likely to attack tin.[44]

Intentional addition of tin salts to food substances does not appear to be common, although protochloride of tin is said sometimes to be added to molasses for the purpose of reducing the color. The chlorides are regarded as more definitely poisonous than other compounds of tin, and for this and other reasons the practice is undesirable. Sanitarians insist that chemical substances likely to be irritating to the human tissues in assimilation or elimination should not be employed in food. Each new irritant, even in small quantity, may add to the burden of organs already weakened by age or previous harsh treatment.

COPPER

Danger is popularly supposed to attend the cooking and especially the long standing of certain foods in copper vessels on account of the verdigris or copper acetate that is sometimes formed, but Professor Long, of the Referee Board of Consulting Scientific Experts,[45] points out that this substance is far less toxic than it was once imagined to be, and he considers it likely that the cases of illness attributed to "verdigris poisoning" reported in the older literature should have been explained in some other way.

The use of copper sulphate for imparting a green color to certain vegetables, such as peas, beans, and asparagus, is a relatively modern practice, having been started in France about 1850. Since the natural green of vegetables is in part destroyed or altered by heat, restoration of the color has appealed to the color sense of some consumers. It must be admitted that this aesthetic gratification is fraught with some degree of danger to health. The experiments by Long show that copper is absorbed and retained in certain tissues, and that even small amounts ingested at brief intervals may have a deleterious action. He concludes that the use of copper salts for coloring foods must be considered as highly objectionable. The United States Government now prohibits the importation of foods colored with copper and also the interstate trade in these substances.

VARIOUS COLORING SUBSTANCES

Copper sulphate is but one of a host of chemical substances applied to various foods for the purpose of altering the color which the foods would otherwise possess. In some cases perhaps it may be the general opinion that by special treatment the attractiveness of a food product is increased, as when dark-colored flour is bleached white with nitrogen peroxide, but in many instances the modification of color is based on preposterously artificial standards. The use of poisonous aniline dyes for staining candies all the colors of the rainbow must be defended, if at all, on aesthetic rather than on sanitary grounds. Some coloring matters in common use, such as the annatto, universally employed in coloring butter, are believed to be without harmful effect, but others are to be viewed with suspicion, and still others, like copper sulphate, are unquestionably dangerous. The whole practice of food coloration at its best involves waste and may entail serious danger to health. Broadly speaking, all modification of the natural color of foodstuffs is based on an idle convention and should be prohibited in the interest of the public welfare. Bleached flour, stained butter, dyed jelly and ice-cream are no whit more desirable as foods than the natural untreated substances; in fact, they are essentially less desirable. If the whole process of food coloration were known to the public, artificially colored foods would not be especially appetizing. Economically the practice is singularly futile. The artificial whitening of flour with the highly poisonous nitrogen peroxide seems hardly worth the extra tax of fifty cents to a dollar a barrel. Such bleaching with a poisonous gas certainly does not improve the nutritive or digestive qualities of flour; it may be insidiously injurious. The solution of the problem of food coloration seems to lie in a policy of educational enlightenment which shall make natural foods appear more desirable than those sold under false colors. Custom, however, buttressed by skilful advertising, offers a difficult barrier to reform in this field.

FOOD PRESERVATIVES

It is not only legitimate, but in every way most desirable, to keep food over from a season of superabundance to a season of scarcity. From time immemorial food has been preserved by drying, smoking, or salting, and, in modern times, by refrigeration and by heat (canning). These latter methods have come to play a large part in the food habits of civilized communities. Since food spoils because of microbic action, all methods of preservation are based upon the destruction of the microbes or the restraint of their growth by various physical and chemical agencies. The use of certain chemical preservatives such as strong sugar and salt solutions, saltpeter brines, and acid pickles has long been known and countenanced. In recent times the employment of chemical preservatives has acquired a new aspect through the increasing tendency of manufacturers to add to food products antiseptic chemicals in wide variety and of dubious physiological effect.

It is not so easy and simple as it might appear to declare that no substance that is poisonous shall be added to food. The scientific conception of a poison is one involving the amount as well as the kind of substance. Common salt itself is poisonous in large doses, but, as everyone knows, small amounts are not only not injurious, but absolutely necessary to health. Well-known and very powerful protoplasmic poisons such as strychnine and quinine are frequently administered in minute doses for medicinal purposes, without causing serious results.

How complicated the question of using food preservatives really is appears in the case of smoked meats and fish, which owe their keeping qualities to the creosote and other substances with which they are impregnated by the smoke. Although these substances are much more highly poisonous than chemical preservatives like benzoic acid, over which much concern has been expressed, but little if any objection has been made to the use of smoked foods.

The use of benzoic acid (benzoate of soda) as a food preservative illustrates several phases of the controversy. Observations by Wiley in 1908 upon so-called "poison squads" were thought by him to indicate that benzoate of soda administered with food led to "a very serious disturbance of the metabolic functions, attended with injury to digestion and health." On the other hand, the experiments of the Referee Board of Scientific Experts (1909), conducted with at least equal care and thoroughness, were considered to warrant the conclusions that:

(1) Sodium benzoate in small doses (under five-tenths of a gram per day)

mixed with the food is without deleterious or poisonous action and is not injurious to health. (2) Sodium benzoate in large doses (up to four grams per day) mixed with the food has not been found to exert any deleterious effect on the general health, nor to act as a poison in the general acceptance of the term. In some directions there were slight modifications in certain physiological processes, the exact significance of which modification is not known. (3) The admixture of sodium benzoate with food in small or large doses has not been found to injuriously affect or impair the quality or nutritive value of such food.

Still later experiments under the auspices of the German government (1913) showed that in the case of dogs and rabbits relatively large doses of benzoic acid (corresponding to sixty to one hundred grams per day for a man weighing one hundred and fifty pounds) were necessary in order to produce demonstrable effects of any kind. This finding may be considered to confirm in a general way the finding of the Referee Board that four grams per day is harmless.

Probably the evidence respecting the effect of benzoic acids and the benzoates when used as food preservatives constitutes as favorable a case as can be made out at the present time for the employment of any chemical substance. Benzoic acid is present in noteworthy amounts in many fruits and berries, especially cranberries, and its presence in these natural foods has never been connected with any injurious action. In point of fact, substances present in many ordinary foodstuffs are converted within the human body first into benzoic acid and then into hippuric acid. Folin's masterly summing up is worth quoting:

We know that the human organism is prepared to take care of and render harmless those small quantities of benzoic acid and benzoic acid compounds which occur in food products or which are formed within the body; we know how this is accomplished and are reasonably sure as to the particular organ which does it. We also know that the mechanism by means of which the poisonous benzoic acid is converted into the harmless hippuric acid is an extremely efficient one, and that it is capable of taking care of relatively enormous quantities of benzoic acid. In this case, as in a great many others, the normal animal organism is abundantly capable of performing the function which it must regularly perform in order to survive. From this point of view it can be argued, and it has been argued with considerable force, that the human organism is abundantly capable of rendering harmless reasonable amounts of benzoic acid or benzoate which are added for purposes of preservation to certain articles of our food. In my opinion this point of view is going to prevail, and the strife will resolve itself into a controversy over how much benzoic acid shall be permitted to go into our daily food.

But we ought to be exceedingly cautious about accepting any definite figure, certainly any large figure, as representing the permissible amount of added benzoic acid in our food. The very fact that we are in possession of an efficient process for converting poisonous benzoic acid into harmless hippuric acid indicates that there is a necessity for doing so. It suggests that even the small quantities of benzoic acid which we get with unadulterated food, or produce within ourselves, might be deleterious to health except for the saving hippuric acid forming process. And because that "factor of safety" is a large one with respect to the normal benzoic acid content of our food it does not follow that we can encroach on it with perfect impunity. What the effect of a general, regular encroachment on it would be cannot be determined by a few relatively short feeding experiments. It is known that while certain chemicals may be taken in substantial quantities for a month or a year without producing demonstrably injurious effects, nevertheless the continued use of the same substances, even in smaller quantities, will eventually undermine the health. Perhaps the final solution of the benzoic acid problem could be best obtained directly from the people at large. If they were to consume benzoic acid as knowingly as they consume, for example, sodic carbonate in soda biscuits, or caffeine and theobromine in coffee and tea, it would not require more than a decade or two before we should have a well-defined and well-founded public opinion on the subject, at least in the medical profession.[46]

With respect to other familiar and more or less poisonous substances used to preserve foods, defense of their harmlessness is far more difficult. Formaldehyde, salicylic acid, sulphurous acid, and sulphite are compounds definitely poisonous in relatively small amounts, their injurious action in minute successive doses in animal experiments is quite marked, and their use in human food products practically without justification. Boric acid and borax are perhaps on a slightly different footing, but are never present in natural foods, and there is no good evidence that their long-continued ingestion in small doses is without injurious effect. It must not be forgotten that all such substances owe their preservative or antiseptic power to the poisonous effect they have upon bacterial protoplasm. It is fair to assume that, in general, bacterial protoplasm is no more easily injured than human protoplasm, and this raises at once the propriety of bringing into repeated contact with human tissues substances likely to produce injury even if such injury is slight and recovery from it is ordinarily easy. In every case the burden of proof should be properly placed on those who advocate the addition of bacterial-restraining substances to food intended for human consumption. It is for them to show that substances powerful enough to hold in check the development of bacteria are yet unable to interfere seriously with the life-processes of the cells of the human body.

When this view of the situation is taken, not only the chemical substances mentioned previously fall under some suspicion, but also certain household preservatives long sanctioned by custom. Spices such as cinnamon, oil of cloves, and the like are, so far as we know, as likely to have an injurious physiological effect when taken in small recurring quantities as are some of the "chemical" preservatives whose use is debarred by law. The chemicals deposited by wood smoke in meat are of a particularly objectionable nature, and their continuous ingestion may quite conceivably lead to serious injury.

One fact persistently comes to the front in any comprehensive study of the food-preservative question, namely, the need of further experiment and observation. We do not at present know what effect is produced in human beings of different ages and varying degrees of strength by the long-continued consumption of food preserved with particular chemicals.

There is, I think, only one way to get at the facts with regard to the various chemicals which have been used for the preservation of foods, and that is by trying them and keeping track of the results. To try them properly, on a sufficiently extensive scale and for a sufficiently long time, is, however, more of a task than can be undertaken by private investigators; for it is only by their continuous use for many years under competent supervision and control that we can hope to attain adequate information for final conclusions. Work of this sort should be done and could very well be done at large government institutions, as, for example, among certain classes of prison inmates. I do not know how many life prisoners or long-term prisoners may be available, but there must be an abundance of them. They would make better subjects than students on whom to try out a substance like boric acid. This, not because they are prisoners whose fate or health is of comparatively little consequence, but because they represent a body of persons whose mode of life is essentially uniform and whose health record could easily be kept for a long period of years. I am well aware that this suggestion will impress many persons as heartless and brutal, but such an experiment would be a mild and humane one when compared with the unrecorded boric acid experiments which have been made by manufacturers on all kinds and conditions of people. Prisoners are unfortunate in not being able to render any useful service to society. Probably not a few would be willing to co-operate in prolonged feeding experiments, similar to the short ones conducted by Dr. Wiley and by the Referee Board. Acceptable reward in the way of well-prepared food of sufficient variety would attract volunteers. If additional inducement were necessary, shortened term of service would probably appeal to many. And in the face of the fact that every civilized country is prepared to sacrifice thousands of its most virile citizens for the honor of its flag (and its foreign trade), the sentiment against endangering the health of a handful of men in the interest of all mankind is not particularly intelligent.[47]

Until such information is forthcoming we do well to err on the side of caution. The desirability of adopting this attitude is especially borne in upon us by the facts already instanced (pp. 2-4) concerning the increased death-rates in the higher-age groups in this country. For aught we now know to the contrary, the relatively high death-rates from degenerative changes in the kidneys, blood vessels, and other organs may be in part caused by the use of irritating chemical substances in food. Although no one chemical by itself and in the quantities in which it is commonly present in food can perhaps be reasonably accused of producing serious and permanent injury, yet when to its effect is superadded the effect of still other poisonous ingredients in spiced, smoked, and preserved foods of all kinds the total burden laid upon the excretory and other organs may be distinctly too great. There can be no escape from the conclusion that the more extensive and widespread the use of preservatives in food the greater the likelihood of injurious consequences to the public health.

The use of spoiled or decomposed food falls under the same head. It cannot be assumed that the irritating substances produced in food by certain kinds of decomposition can be continually consumed with impunity. We do not even know whether these decomposition products may not be more fundamentally injurious than preservatives that might be added to prevent decomposition!

So far as our present knowledge indicates, therefore, effort should be directed (1) to the purveying of food as far as possible in a fresh condition; (2) to the avoidance of chemical preservatives of all kinds except those unequivocally demonstrated to be harmless. The methods of preserving food by drying, by refrigeration, and by heating and sealing are justified by experience as well as on theoretical grounds, and the same statement can be made regarding the use of salt and sugar solutions. But the use of sulphites in sausage and chopped meat, the addition of formaldehyde to milk, and of boric acid or sodium fluoride to butter are practices altogether objectionable from the standpoint of public health.

The remedy is obvious and has been frequently suggested--namely, laws prohibiting the addition of any chemical to food except in certain definitely specified cases. The presumption then would be--as in truth it is--that such chemicals are more or less dangerous, and proof of innocuousness must be brought forward before any one substance can be listed as an exception to the general rule. Such laws would include not only the use of chemicals or preservatives, but the employment of substances to "improve the appearance" of foodstuffs. As already pointed out, the childish practice of artificially coloring foods involves waste and sometimes danger. It rests on no deep-seated human need; food that is natural and untampered with may be made the fashion just as easily as the color and cut of clothing are altered by the fashion-monger. The incorporation of any chemical substance into food for preservative or cosmetic purposes could wisely be subject to a general prohibition, and the necessary list of exceptions (substances such as sugar and salt) should be passed on by a national board of experts or by some authoritative organization like the American Public Health Association.

FOOD SUBSTITUTES

On grounds of economy or convenience familiar and natural articles of food are sometimes replaced or supplemented by artificial chemical products, or by substances whose food value is not so definitely established. I need refer only briefly to those notorious instances of adulteration in which chicory is added to coffee, or ground olive stones to pepper, or glucose to candy. On hygienic grounds alone some such practices are not open to criticism, however fraudulent they may be from the standpoint of public morals. It might be argued with some plausibility that chicory is not so likely to harm the human organism as caffeine and that sprinklings of ground cocoanut shell are more wholesome than pepper. But there is another group of cases in which the artificial substitute is strictly objectionable. The use of the coal-tar product saccharin for sweetening purposes is an example. This substance, whose sweetening power is five hundred times as great as that of cane sugar, has no nutritive value in the quantities in which it would be consumed, and in not very large quantities (over 0.3 gram per day) is likely to induce disturbance of digestion. As a substitute for sugar in ordinary foodstuffs it is undesirable.[48]

The use of cheap chemically prepared flavors such as "fruit ethers" in "soft drinks," fruit syrups, and the like in place of the more expensive natural fruit extracts affords another well-known instance of substitution. Probably more important hygienically is the production of "foam" in "soda water" by saponin, a substance known to be injurious for red blood corpuscles.

Among the many other familiar examples of food substitution, sophistication, and adulteration there are some of demonstrable hygienic disadvantage and others whose chief demerit lies in simple deception. Of practically all it may be said that they are indefensible from the standpoint of public policy since they are based on the intent to make foodstuffs appear other than what they really are.

It is the opinion of some who have closely followed the course of food adulteration that, while the amount of general sophistication--legally permissible and otherwise--has greatly increased in recent years, the proportion of really injurious adulteration has fallen off. Be that as it may, it is plain that the opportunity for wholesale experimentation with new substances should not be allowed to rest without control in the hands of manufacturers and dealers largely impelled by commercial motives. So long as the motive of gain is allowed free scope, so long will a small minority of unscrupulous persons add cheap, inferior, and sometimes dangerous ingredients to foodstuffs. The net of restriction must be drawn tighter and tighter. The motives leading to the tampering with food fall mainly under three heads: (1) a desire to preserve food from spoiling or deterioration; (2) a puerile fancy--often skilfully fostered for mercenary reasons--for a conventional appearance, as for polished rice, bleached flour, and grass-green peas; and (3) intent to make the less valuable appear more valuable--deliberate fraud. Only the first-named motive can claim any legitimate justification, and its gratification by the use of chemical preservatives is surrounded with hygienic difficulties and uncertainty, as already set forth. From the unbiased view of human physiology the dangers of slow poisoning from chemically treated foods must be regarded as no less real because they are insidious and not easily traced.

FOOTNOTES:

[32] E. S. Reynolds, Lancet, I (1901), 166.

[33] The sulphuric acid used in making glucose in the United States is authoritatively declared to be absolutely free from arsenic (report of hearing before Illinois State Food Standard Commission, June 21-23, 1916; see Amer. Food Jour., July, 1916, p. 315).

[34] E. W. Miller, Jour. Home Economics, VIII (1916), 361.

[35] Phelps and Stevenson, Hyg. Lab., U.S. Public Health Service, Bull. 96, 1914, p. 55.

[36] Harrington and Richardson, Manual of Practical Hygiene, 5th ed., p. 224.

[37] See Alice Hamilton, "Hygiene of the Painters' Trade," U.S. Bureau of Labor Statistics, Bull. 120, 1913.

[38] In 1909 the value of foods canned in the United States amounted to about $300,000,000 (U.S. Dept. of Agric., Bull. 196, 1915).

[39] W. D. Bigelow, Amer. Food Jour., XI (1916), 461.

[40] Arch. f. Hyg., XLV (1902), 88; ibid., LXIII (1907), 67.

[41] See, e.g., Harrington and Richardson, Practical Hygiene, 5th ed., p. 274.

[42] Ztschr. f. Hyg., LXXV-LXXVI (1913-14), 55.

[43] Bigelow, loc. cit.

[44] A. W. Bitting, U.S. Dept. of Agric., Bull. 196, 1915.

[45] U.S. Dept. of Agric., Report 97, 1913.

[46] Folin, Preservatives and Other Chemicals in Foods (Harvard University Press, 1914), p. 32.

[47] Folin, op. cit., p. 42.

[48] See U.S. Dept. of Agric., Report 94, 1911.

CHAPTER V

FOOD-BORNE PATHOGENIC BACTERIA

Many cases of so-called food poisoning are due to the presence of pathogenic bacteria in the food. In some instances, as in the typical meat poisoning epidemics, symptoms develop so soon after eating that the particular food involved is immediately suspected and laid hands on. In other cases the guilty article of food is difficult to trace. Certain cases of tuberculosis are undoubtedly caused by swallowing tubercle bacilli in the food, but the precise source and date of infection can be rarely, if ever, certainly established.

The presence of pathogenic bacteria in food is usually due either to the contamination of the food by infected human beings during the process of preparation or serving, or to an infection of the animal from which the food is derived. The relative importance of these two factors is quite different in the various infections.

TYPHOID FOOD INFECTION

The typhoid bacillus does not attack any of the domestic animals;

consequently all food-borne typhoid is caused more or less directly by human contamination. A remarkable instance of typhoid infection due to food was reported in 1914 in Hanford, California, where ninety-three typhoid cases were caused by eating Spanish spaghetti served at a public dinner.[49] Investigation showed that this dish was prepared by a woman typhoid-carrier who was harboring living typhoid bacilli at the time she mixed the sauce for the spaghetti before baking. Further laboratory experiments indicated that the ordinary baking temperature at which the spaghetti was cooked was not only not sufficient to sterilize the food, but afforded a favorable opportunity for the bacteria in the interior of the mass to multiply. The infection of the food was consequently heavy and involved a very large proportion (57 per cent) of those present at the dinner.

Merited celebrity attaches to the exploits of the typhoid-carrier, Mary Malloy, who, in pursuing her career as cook in and about New York City, is known to have caused at least seven typhoid outbreaks in various families in which she worked and one extensive hospital epidemic. Similar cases of typhoid food infection by employees in restaurants and public institutions are by no means uncommon, and show the necessity of protecting food from contamination during the whole process of preparation and serving. Acting on this principle, the Department of Health of New York City has inaugurated a comprehensive examination of the cooks and waiters (approximately 90,000) employed in the public restaurants and dining-rooms in that city. Results have been obtained in the discovery of typhoid-carriers and of cases of communicable disease that amply justify this procedure as an important measure for protecting the community against the dissemination of infection.

Some foods by their origin are exposed more than others to typhoid contamination. Such vegetables as lettuce, celery, radishes, and watercress, which are commonly eaten without cooking, are more likely to convey typhoid than peas, beans, and potatoes. A typhoid outbreak apparently due to watercress has been reported from Philadelphia.[50] At a wedding breakfast to forty-three guests on June 24, 1913, watercress sandwiches were served, and subsequent inquiry showed that nineteen of the guests partook of these sandwiches. Eighteen of this number became ill with typhoid fever within a month, the illness developing in most cases after the guests had scattered to their summer homes. Those who did not eat watercress sandwiches were not affected. Typhoid infection by uncooked celery has also been reported.[51]

The practice of using human excreta as fertilizer in truck gardens is sometimes responsible for a dangerous contamination of the soil, which is communicated to the growing plants and persists for a long time.[52] Even scrupulous washing of vegetables is not sufficient to render them bacterially clean. In the future the danger to the community from this source is likely to become increasingly serious unless the growing use of this method of soil enrichment is definitely checked.

In 1915 an increasing number of typhoid cases in South Philadelphia led to an investigation by the state health department.[53] This disclosed the fact that the majority of the cases were clustered in and about three public markets.

These are all curb markets--fruits, vegetables, pastry, clothing, and miscellaneous merchandise of every description are dumped on push-carts and pavements without regard for any sanitary precautions. The patrons of these markets handle and pick over the exposed foodstuffs, thus giving every opportunity for the transmission of disease....

The greatest number of cases occurred in the immediate vicinity of the Christian Street Market. This market is largely patronized by the inhabitants of the section known as "Little Italy." The patrons of the South Street Market are principally Hebrews, while the Seventh Street Market is patronized in the main by Hebrews and Poles.

The following conclusion was reached regarding the particularly large number of cases among persons of one nationality:

Our inspectors have found that the different methods used by the Italians and Hebrews in the preparation of their food are responsible for the larger number of cases being found in the vicinity of the Christian Street Market in Little Italy. It is the custom of the Italians to eat many of the fruits and vegetables raw, while the Hebrews cook the greater portion of their food. It is presumably due to this custom that the members of the Italian colony have suffered to a greater extent than the other residents of the district.

A bacterial examination of various kinds of vegetables obtained from push-carts and curb markets led to the finding of the typhoid bacillus upon some of the celery. It would naturally be difficult to determine in such cases whether the typhoid bacilli were derived from infected soil in which the celery was grown or whether the contamination occurred through improper handling.

Bread, when marketed unwrapped, is subject to contamination from flies and from uncleanly handling. Katherine Howell[54] has shown that unwrapped loaves of bread sold in Chicago were more or less thickly smeared with bacteria and were coated on the average with a much larger number than wrapped loaves. In some cases typhoid fever has been directly traced to bread. Hinton[55] has recorded the occurrence of seven typhoid cases in the Elgin (Illinois) State Hospital, which were apparently due to a typhoid-carrier whose duty it was as attendant to slice the bread before serving. When this typhoid-bearing attendant was transferred to another department where she handled no uncooked food, cases of typhoid ceased to appear.[56]

Food such as milk that is not only eaten customarily without cooking, but is also suitable for the growth of typhoid bacilli, needs to be particularly safeguarded. It is noteworthy that the compulsory pasteurization of milk in New York, Chicago, and other large American cities has been accompanied by a great diminution in the prevalence of typhoid fever. Until recent years milk-borne typhoid in the United States has been common and hundreds of typhoid epidemics have been traced to this source.

One food animal, the oyster, frequently eaten raw, has been connected on good evidence with certain typhoid outbreaks.[57] The number of well-established oyster typhoid epidemics is not great, however, and the danger from this source has sometimes been exaggerated. The source of oyster contamination is in sewage pollution either of the shellfish beds or of the brackish water in which the oyster is sometimes placed to "fatten" before it is marketed. State and federal supervision of the oyster industry in the United States in recent years has largely done away with the taking of oysters from infected waters, and although oysters--and clams and mussels as well--must be steadily safeguarded against sewage contamination, the actual occurrence of oyster infection at the present time is believed to be relatively rare.

Probably the most effective method of preventing typhoid food infection is to investigate every case of typhoid fever and trace it, so far as practicable, to its origin. In this way typhoid-carriers may be discovered and other foci of infection brought to light. Carriers, once found, may be given proper advice and warned that they constitute a danger to others; the complete control of typhoid-carriers who are not disposed to act as advised is a difficult problem and one not yet solved by public health authorities.

ASIATIC CHOLERA

With Asiatic cholera, just as with typhoid fever, domestic animals are not susceptible to the disease, all cases of infection having a direct human origin. Drinking-water is the usual vehicle of cholera infection, and even in countries where the disease Is endemic, food-borne outbreaks of this disease are far less common than those of typhoid fever. Occasional instances of Asiatic cholera due to milk supply and to contaminated fruits or lettuce are on record, but these are exceptional and cannot be regarded as exemplifying a common mode of spread of this disease. The extent, however, to which dwellers in tropical countries--and indeed in all lands--are at the mercy of their household helpers is illustrated by the following experience of the English bacteriologist, Hankin. "I have seen," he says, "a cook cooling a jelly by standing it in a small irrigation ditch that ran in front of his cookhouse. The water running in this drain came from a well in which I had detected the cholera microbe. He cleaned a spoon by dipping it in the drain and rubbing it with his fingers; then he used it to stir the jelly."[58]

TUBERCULOSIS

Animal experiments have shown that both meat and milk derived from tuberculous cattle are capable of conveying infection. The precise degree of danger to human beings from the use of these foods under modern conditions is still in dispute. Since the tubercle bacillus of bovine origin differs from the tubercle bacillus of human origin in certain well-defined particulars, it is possible by careful study to distinguish the human infections caused by the bovine bacillus from those caused by the so-called human tubercle bacillus. Additional comparative investigations are needed in this field, and these may enable us to estimate eventually more fully than is possible at present the extent of human tuberculous infection derived from bovine sources.

Meat is a less likely source of infection than milk, chiefly because it is rarely eaten without cooking. Opinion regarding the actual frequency of the transmission of tuberculosis by means of the meat of tuberculous cattle has been widely at variance in the past, and must even now be based on indirect evidence. There is no well-established instance of human infection from the use of the flesh of tuberculous cattle. The significance of this fact, however, is diminished by the observation that tubercle bacilli can pass through the intestinal wall without leaving any trace of their passage and can make their way to the lungs or to other distant organs where they find opportunity for growth. This, together with the long period which usually elapses between the actual occurrence of infection and the discovery of the existence of infection, makes the difficulty of securing valid evidence peculiarly great. Opposed to any very frequent occurrence of meat-borne tuberculosis are the facts that the tubercle bacillus is not commonly or abundantly present in the masses of muscle usually marketed as "meat," that the tubercle germ itself is not a spore-bearer and is killed by ordinary cooking, and that the reported cases of the finding of tubercle bacilli of bovine origin in adults over sixteen years of age are extremely rare. This latter fact is perhaps the strongest evidence indicating that tuberculous meat infection, although theoretically possible, is at least not of common occurrence.

Most of the commissions and official agencies that have considered the precautions to be taken against possible tuberculous meat infection are agreed that the entire carcass of an animal should be condemned when the tuberculous lesions are generalized or when the lesions are extensive in one or both body cavities as well as when the lesions are "multiple, acute, and actively progressive." Any organ showing evidence of tuberculous lesions is obviously not to be passed as food. On the other hand, it is considered that portions of properly inspected animals may be put on the market if the tuberculous lesion is local and limited and the main part of the body is unaffected; in such cases contamination of the meat in dressing must be avoided. It is the general belief that when such precautionary measures are taken the danger of tuberculous infection through properly cooked meat is so slight as to be negligible.

Milk is a much more likely vehicle than meat for the transmission of tuberculosis. Freshly drawn raw milk from tuberculous cattle may contain enormous numbers of tubercle bacilli, especially if the udder is diseased. Contamination of milk by the manure of tuberculous cows can also occur. Observers in England, Germany, France, and the United States have found tubercle bacilli in varying numbers in market milk, and have proved that such milk is infectious for laboratory animals. Although, as pointed out with reference to meat infection, the difficulties of tracing any particular case of tuberculosis to its source are very great, there are a number of instances on record in which the circumstantial evidence strongly indicates that milk was the vehicle of infection. Especially convincing are the observations on the relative frequency of infection with bovine and human tubercle bacilli at different ages as shown in the following tabulation:[59]

===

=====	Adults Sixteen Years Old and Over	Children Five to Sixteen Years Old	Children under Five Years
Human tubercle bacilli found	677	99	161
Bovine tubercle bacilli found	9	33	59

The large proportion of bovine tubercle bacillus infections in children stands in all probability in causal relation to the relatively extensive use of raw milk in the child's dietary.

The proper pasteurization of milk affords a safe and reasonably satisfactory means of preventing tuberculous infection from this source. The general introduction of the pasteurizing process in most American cities has ample justification from the standpoint of the prevention of infection.

VARIOUS MILK-BORNE INFECTIONS

The facts related in the foregoing pages indicate that of all foods milk is the most likely to convey disease germs into the human body. This is partly due to the fact that milk is sometimes obtained from diseased animals, and partly to the fact that unless great care is taken it may readily become contaminated during the process of collection and transportation; if milk is once seeded with dangerous bacteria these can multiply in the excellent culture medium it affords. It is also partly because milk is commonly taken into the alimentary tract without being cooked. For these reasons the amount of illness traceable to raw milk far exceeds that ascribable to any other food.

There are several infections that may be communicated by milk, but are rarely if ever due to other foodstuffs. Diphtheria and scarlet fever are perhaps the best known of these. Both diseases have been repeatedly traced to the use of particular milk supplies, although various forms of individual contact also play a large role in their dissemination. Milk-borne scarlet fever and diphtheria seem to be generally, if not always, due to the direct contamination of the milk from human sources. It is considered possible, however, by some investigators that the cow may sometimes become infected from human sources with the virus of scarlet fever or diphtheria and may herself occasionally contribute directly to the infection of the milk.

A serious milk-borne disease, which has lately been conspicuous in Boston, Chicago, Baltimore, and other American cities under the name of "septic sore throat" or "streptococcus sore throat," originates apparently in some cases from infection of the udder of the cow by an infected milker; in other cases the milk has seemingly been directly infected by a human "carrier." The specific germ is thought to have been isolated and its connection with the disease demonstrated in the laboratory. This disease, like diphtheria and scarlet fever, is sometimes due to contact. It is not known to be caused by any food except milk.

Foot-and-mouth disease of cattle is transmissible to man through the milk of infected cattle, but this infection in man is not very common or as a rule very serious. So far as known, it is not communicated to man in any other way except through the use of uncooked milk.

Such cases of infection or "poisoning" by milk may be prevented, as already stated, by the exclusive use of heated milk. The possible occurrence of nutritional disturbances (e.g., scurvy) in a small proportion of the children fed on pasteurized or boiled milk is considered by many physicians to be easily remedied and to possess much less practical importance than the avoidance of infection.

POSSIBLE INFECTION WITH B. PROTEUS

One widely distributed organism known as Bacillus proteus has been several times held responsible for food poisoning outbreaks, but it is not yet certain how far this accusation is justified. B. proteus is related to B. coli, but most varieties do not ferment lactose and are much more actively proteolytic than the latter organism, as shown by their ability to liquefy gelatin and casein.

Like B. coli, they form indol and ferment dextrose with gas production. Varieties of B. proteus are found widely distributed in decomposing organic matter of all sorts.

The evidence upon which this bacillus is regarded as the cause of food poisoning is not altogether convincing. The outbreak described by Pfuhl[60] is typical. Eighty-one soldiers in a garrison at Hanover were suddenly attacked with acute gastro-enteritis four to twelve hours after eating sausage meat. The meat was found to contain B. proteus in large numbers, although it was prepared with ordinary care and was entirely normal in appearance, taste, and smell. Rats and mice fed with the sausage became ill and B. proteus was isolated from the blood and internal organs. But these animals sometimes die when fed with quite normal meat, and B. proteus and other common intestinal bacteria are often isolated from the body after death. B. proteus, in fact, is found in many animal foods and in the apparently normal human intestine. Like B. coli, it frequently invades the internal organs after or shortly before death. Finding B. proteus in food or in the internal organs does not therefore constitute definite proof of any causal relationship. The evidence attributing other outbreaks to infection with B. proteus is similarly inconclusive.

It is equally uncertain whether the production of a poison in food by this species can in any degree be held responsible for meat poisoning. B. proteus is common enough in decomposing food material and under certain circumstances is known to generate substances that are toxic for man. It is possibly true that toxic substances are produced in the early stages of decomposition by this organism. In the opinion of Mandel[61] and others, if any injurious effect at all is to be attributed to B. proteus, it is in the nature of an intoxication and not an infection (see chapter viii). So far as the existing evidence goes, the question of the responsibility of this organism for food poisoning is still an open one.

FOOTNOTES:

[49] Sawyer, Jour. Amer. Med. Assoc., LXIII (1914), 1537.

[50] Eng. News, LXX (1913), 322.

[51] Morse, Report of State Board of Health of Mass., 1899, p. 761.

[52] R. H. Creel, Reprint from Public Health Reports, No. 72, Washington, 1912.

[53] Health Bull. No. 76, Pennsylvania State Department of Health, December, 1915.

[54] Amer. Jour. Public Health, II (1912), 321.

[55] Institution Quarterly, III (1912), 18.

[56] See also a similar instance reported by Lumsden, Hyg. Lab., U.S. Public Health and Marine Hosp. Service, Bull. 78, p. 165.

[57] For a discussion of the oyster question see G. W. Fuller, Jour. of Franklin Institute, August, 1905; N.Y. City Dept. of Health, Monthly Bull., November, 1913, and May, 1915; H. S. Cumming, U.S. Public Health Service, Pub. Health Bull. 74, March, 1916.

[58] Lancet, II (1895), 4G.

[59] Park and Krumwiede, Jour. Med. Research, N.S., XVIII (1910), 363.

[60] Ztschr. f. Hyg., XXXV (1900), 265.

[61] Centralbl. f. Bakt., I, Orig., LXVI (1912), 194.

CHAPTER VI

FOOD-BORNE PATHOGENIC BACTERIA (Continued)

PARATYPHOID INFECTION

The most characteristic examples of "food poisoning," popularly speaking, are those in which the symptoms appear shortly after eating and in which gastro-intestinal disturbances predominate. In the typical group-outbreaks of this sort all grades of severity are manifested, but as a rule recovery takes place. The great majority of such cases that have been investigated by modern bacteriological methods show the presence of bacilli belonging to the so-called paratyphoid group (B. paratyphosus or B. enteritidis). Especially is it true of meat poisoning epidemics that paratyphoid bacilli are found in causal relation with them. Hener[62] enumerates forty-two meat poisoning outbreaks in Germany in which bacilli of this group were shown to be implicated, and Savage[63] gives a list of twenty-seven similar outbreaks in Great Britain. In the United States relatively few outbreaks of this character have been placed on record, but it cannot be assumed that this is due to their rarity, since no adequate investigation of food poisoning cases is generally carried out in our American communities.

Typical paratyphoid outbreaks.--Kaensche[64] describes an outbreak at Breslau involving over eighty persons in which chopped beef was apparently the bearer of infection. The animal from which the meat came had been ill with severe diarrhea and high fever and was slaughtered as an emergency measure (notgeschlachtet). On examination a pathological condition of the liver and other organs was noted by a veterinarian who declared the meat unfit for use and ordered it destroyed. It was, however, stolen, carried secretly to Breslau, and portions of it were distributed to different sausage-makers, who sold it for the most part as hamburger steak (Hackfleisch). The meat itself presented nothing abnormal in color, odor, or consistency. Nevertheless, illness followed in some cases after the use of very small portions. With some of those affected the symptoms were very severe, but there were no deaths. Bacilli of the Bacillus enteritidis type were isolated from the meat.

A large and unusually severe outbreak reported by McWeeney[65] occurred in November, 1908, among the inmates of an industrial school for girls at Limerick, Ireland. There were 73 cases with 9 deaths out of the total number of 197 pupils. The brunt of the attack fell on the first or Senior class comprising 67 girls between the ages of thirteen and seventeen. Out of 55 girls belonging to this class who partook of beef stew for dinner 53 sickened, and 8 of these died. One of the two who were not affected ate the gravy and potatoes but not the beef. Some of the implicated beef was also eaten as cold meat by girls in some of the other classes, and also caused illness. Part of the meat had been eaten previously without producing any ill effects. "The escape of those who partook of portions of the same carcass on October 27 and 29 [five days earlier] may be accounted for either by unequal distribution of the virus, or by thorough cooking which destroyed it. Some of the infective material must, however, have escaped the roasting of the 29th, and, multiplying rapidly, have rendered the whole piece intensely toxic and infective during the five days that elapsed before the fatal Tuesday when it was finally consumed." The animal from which the fore quarter of the beef was taken had been privately slaughtered by a local butcher. No reliable information could be obtained about the condition of the calf at, or slightly prior to, slaughter. The meat, however, was sold at so low a price that it was evidently not regarded as of prime quality. In this outbreak the agglutination reactions of the blood of the patients and the characteristics of the bacilli isolated showed the infection to be due to a typical strain of Bacillus enteritidis.

An epidemic of food poisoning occurred in July, 1915, at and near Westerly, Rhode Island.[66] The outbreak was characterized by the usual symptoms of acute gastro-enteritis, and followed the eating of pie which was obtained at a restaurant in Westerly. All the circumstances of the outbreak showed that a particular batch of pies was responsible. About sixty persons were made seriously ill and four died. There was no unusual taste or odor to the pies to excite suspicion. The symptoms followed the eating of various kinds of pie: custard, squash, lemon, chocolate, apple, etc., that had been made with the same pie-crust mixture. Bacillus paratyphosus B was isolated from samples of pie that were examined. No definite clue was obtained as to the exact source of infection of the pie mixture. It is possible that the pie became infected in the restaurant through the agency of a paratyphoid-carrier, but since there had been no change in the personnel of the restaurant for several months, this explanation is largely conjectural. Possibly some ingredient of animal origin was primarily infected.

General characters of paratyphoid infection.--The symptoms of paratyphoid food infection are varied. As a rule the first signs of trouble appear within six to twelve hours after eating, but sometimes they may come on within half an hour, or they may not appear until after twenty-four to forty-eight hours. Gastro-intestinal irritation is practically always present, and may take the form of a mild "indigestion" or slight diarrhea or may be of great severity accompanied with agonizing abdominal pain. Fever is usual, but is generally not very high. Recovery may occur quickly, so that within two or three days the patient regains his normal state, or it may be very slow, so that the effects of the attack linger for weeks or months.

Investigators have noted the occurrence of at least two clinical types of paratyphoid infection, the commoner gastro-intestinal type just described and a second type resembling typhoid fever very closely, and occasionally not to be distinguished from it except by careful bacterial examination. It is not yet clear how these two clinical varieties are related to the amount and nature of the infecting food material. No difference in the type of paratyphoid bacillus has been observed to be associated with the difference in clinical manifestation. Possibly the amount of toxin present in the food eaten as well as the number of bacilli may exercise some influence. The individual idiosyncrasy of the patient doubtless plays a part.

While there is still some uncertainty about particular features of paratyphoid infection, a few significant facts have been clearly established: (1) Certain articles of diet are much more commonly associated than others with this type of food poisoning. The majority of recorded outbreaks are connected with the use of meat, milk, fish, and other protein foods. Vegetables and cereals have been less commonly implicated, fruits rarely. (2) In many, though not all, of the cases of paratyphoid meat poisoning it has been demonstrated that the meat concerned has been derived from an animal slaughtered while ailing (notgeschlachtet, to use the expressive German term). There seems reason to believe that in such an animal, "killed to save its life," the specific paratyphoid germ is present as an infection before death. Milk also has caused paratyphoid poisoning and in certain of these cases has been found to be derived from a cow suffering from enteritis or some other disorder. (3) There is evidence that originally wholesome food may become infected with paratyphoid bacilli during the process of preparation or serving in precisely the same way that it may become infected with typhoid bacilli; the handling of the food by a paratyphoid-carrier is commonly responsible for this. In a few instances the disease is passed on from case to case, but this mode of infection seems exceedingly rare and is not nearly so frequent as "contact" infection in typhoid. (4) The majority of paratyphoid outbreaks are associated with the use of uncooked or partly cooked food. A selective action is often manifested, those persons who have eaten the incriminated food substance raw or imperfectly cooked being most seriously affected, while those who have partaken of the same food after cooking remain exempt.

The discovery of the connection of paratyphoid bacilli with meat poisoning dates from the investigation by Gartner,[67] in 1888, of a meat poisoning outbreak In Frankenhausen, a small town in Germany. This epidemic was traced to the use of meat from a cow that was slaughtered because she was ill with a severe enteritis. Fifty-eight persons were affected in varying grades of severity; the attack resulted fatally in one young workman who ate about eight hundred grams of raw meat. Gartner isolated from the spleen of the fatal case and also from the flesh and intestines of the cow a bacillus to which he gave the name B. enteritidis. Inoculation experiments showed it to be pathogenic for a number of animal species. Bacilli with similar characters have since been isolated in a number of other meat poisoning epidemics in Germany, Belgium, France, and England. One well-studied instance of food poisoning due to the paratyphoid bacillus has been reported in the United States.[68]

The bacteria of the paratyphoid group are closely related to the true typhoid bacillus, but differ from the latter organism in being able to ferment glucose with gas production. They are more highly pathogenic for the lower animals than is the typhoid bacillus, but apparently somewhat less pathogenic for man. Most types of paratyphoid bacilli found in food poisoning produce more or less rapidly a considerable amount of alkali, and, if they are inoculated into milk containing a few drops of litmus, the milk after a time becomes a deep blue color. Several distinct varieties of paratyphoid bacilli have been discovered. The main differences shown by these varieties are agglutinative differences. That is, the blood serum of an animal that has been inoculated with a particular culture or strain will agglutinate that strain and also other strains isolated from certain other meat poisoning epidemics, but will not agglutinate certain culturally similar paratyphoid bacteria found in connection with yet other outbreaks. Except in this single matter of agglutination reaction, no constant distinction between these varieties has been demonstrated. The clinical features of the infections produced in man and in the higher animals by the different varieties seem to be very similar if not identical.

The bacillus discovered by Gartner (loc. cit.) and known as B. enteritidis or Gartner's bacillus is commonly taken as the type of one of the agglutinative varieties. Bacilli with all the characters of Gartner's bacillus have been found in meat poisoning epidemics in various places in Belgium and Germany. Mayer[69] has compiled a list of forty-eight food poisoning outbreaks occurring between 1888 and 1911 and attributed to B. enteritidis Gartner. These outbreaks comprised approximately two thousand cases and twenty deaths. In twenty-three of the forty-eight outbreaks the meat was derived from animals known to be ill at the time, or shortly before, they were slaughtered. Sausage and chopped meat of undetermined origin were responsible for eleven of the remaining twenty-five outbreaks. Two of the B. enteritidis outbreaks were attributed to Vanille Pudding; one, to potato salad.

In other food poisoning outbreaks a bacillus is found which is culturally similar to the Gartner bacillus, but refuses to agglutinate with the Gartner bacillus serum. Its cultural and agglutination reactions are almost, if not quite, identical with those of the bacilli found in human cases of paratyphoid fever which have no known connection with food poisoning. Mayer[70] gives a list of seventy-seven outbreaks of food poisoning (1893-1911) in which organisms variously designated as "B. paratyphosus B" or as "B. suipestifer" were held to be responsible. The total number of cases (two thousand) and deaths (twenty) is about the same as ascribed to B. enteritidis. According to Mayer's tabulation meat from animals definitely known to be ailing is less commonly implicated in this type (ten in seventy-seven) than in B. enteritidis outbreaks (twenty-three in forty-eight). Sausage and chopped meat of unknown origin, however, were connected with eighteen outbreaks.

The bacillus named B. suipestifer was formerly believed to be the cause of hog cholera, but it is now thought to be merely a secondary invader in this disease; it is identical with the bacillus called B. paratyphosus B in its cultural and to a large extent in its agglutinative behavior, but is regarded by some investigators as separable from the latter on the basis of particularly delicate discriminatory tests. Bainbridge, Savage, and other English investigators consider indeed that the true food poisoning cases should be ascribed to B. suipestifer and would restrict the term B. paratyphosus to those bacteria causing "an illness clinically indistinguishable from typhoid fever." German investigators, on the other hand, regard B. suipestifer and B. paratyphosus B as identical. My own investigations[71] indicate that there is a real distinction between these two types.

Bearing directly on this question is the discussion concerning the distribution of the food poisoning bacilli in nature. Most investigators in Germany, where the majority of food poisoning outbreaks have occurred, or at least have been bacteriologically studied, are of the opinion that B. suipestifer (the same in their opinion as B. paratyphosus B) is much more widely distributed than B. enteritidis and that it occurs, especially in certain regions, as in the southern part of the German Empire, quite commonly in the intestinal tract of healthy human beings. Such paratyphoid-carriers, it is supposed, may contaminate food through handling or preparation just as typhoid-carriers are known to do. A number of outbreaks in which contamination of food during preparation is thought to have occurred have been reported by Jacobitz and Kayser[72] (vermicelli), Reinhold[73] (fish), and others. Reinhold notes that in one outbreak several persons who had nursed those who were ill became ill themselves, indicating possible contact infection. In another outbreak also reported by Reinhold it was observed that those who partook of the infected food, in this case dried codfish, on the first day were not so severely affected as those who ate what was left over on the second day. A bacillus belonging to the paratyphoid group was isolated from the stools of patients, but not from the dried codfish. These facts were interpreted as signifying that the fish had become infected in the process of preparation and that the bacilli multiplied in the food while it was standing.

There seems no doubt that certain cases of paratyphoid food poisoning are caused by contamination of the food during preparation and are, sometimes at least, due to infection by human carriers. The bacilli in such cases are usually (according to many German investigators) or always (according to most English bacteriologists) of the B. suipestifer type. Other cases are due to pathogenic bacteria derived from diseased animals, and these bacteria are often, possibly always, of a slightly different character (B. enteritidis Gartner). It is still unsettled whether both types of food poisoning bacteria are always associated with disease processes of man or animals, or whether they are organisms of wide distribution which may at times acquire pathogenic properties. In certain regions, as in North Germany and England, such bacteria are rarely, if ever, found except in connection with definite cases of disease. In parts of Southwest Germany, on the other hand, they are said to occur with extraordinary frequency in the intestines of healthy men and animals. Savage[74] believes that there is some confusion on this subject owing to the existence of saprophytic bacteria which he calls "Paragaertner" forms and which bear a close resemblance to the "true" Gartner bacilli. They can be distinguished from the latter only by an extended series of tests. The bacilli of this group show remarkable variability, and in the opinion of some investigators "mutations" sometimes occur which lead to the transformation of one type into another.[75]

In spite of the present uncertainty regarding the relationship and significance of the varieties observed, a few facts emerge plainly from the confusion: (1) The majority of meat poisoning outbreaks that have been bacterially studied in recent years have been traceable to one or another member of this group and not to "ptomain poisoning." (2) Bacteria of the paratyphoid enteritidis group that are culturally alike but agglutinatively dissimilar can, when taken in with the food, give rise to identical clinical symptoms in man. (3) Food poisoning bacteria of this group, when derived directly from diseased animals, seem more likely to be of the Gartner type (B. enteritidis) than of the B. suipestifer type.

Toxin production.--The problem of the production of toxin by the bacteria of this group and the possible relation of the toxin to food poisoning has been much discussed. Broth cultures in which the living bacilli have been destroyed by heat or from which they have been removed by filtration contain a soluble poison. When this germ-free broth is injected into mice, guinea-pigs, or rabbits, the animals die from the effects. Practically nothing is known about the nature of the poisonous substances concerned, except that they are heat-resistant. They are probably not to be classed with the so-called true toxins generated by the diphtheria and tetanus bacilli, since there is no evidence that they give rise to antibodies when injected into susceptible animals. In the opinion of some investigators the formation of these toxic bodies by the paratyphoid-enteritidis bacilli in meat and other protein foodstuffs is responsible for certain outbreaks and also for some of the phenomena of food poisoning, the rapid development of symptoms being regarded as due to the ingested poisons, whereas the later manifestations are considered those of a true infection. Opposed to this view is the fact that well-cooked food has proved distinctly less liable to cause food poisoning than raw or imperfectly cooked food.

A large proportion of the recorded meat poisoning outbreaks are significantly due to sausages made from raw meat and to meat pies, puddings, and jellies. This is most likely because the heat used in cooking such foods is insufficient to produce germicidal results. In milk-borne epidemics also it is noteworthy that the users of raw milk are the ones affected. For example, respecting an extensive B. enteritidis outbreak in and about Newcastle, England, it is stated:

In no instance was a person who had used only boiled milk known to have been affected. Thus in one family, consisting of husband, wife, and wife's mother, the two women drank a small quantity of raw milk from the farm, at the most a tumblerful, and both were taken ill about twelve hours later. The husband, on the other hand, habitually drank a pint a day, but always boiled. He followed his usual custom on this occasion, and was unaffected.[76]

When in addition it is taken into consideration that the ordinary roasting or broiling of a piece of meat is often not sufficient to produce a germicidal temperature throughout, the argument that a heat-resistant toxin is present in such cases is not conclusive. It must be remembered also that in some outbreaks those persons consuming raw or partly cooked meat have been affected while at the same time others eating well-cooked meat from the same animal have remained exempt; this would seem to indicate the destruction of living bacilli by heat, since the toxic substances formed by these organisms are heat-resistant. The view that a definite infection occurs, is favored, too, by the fact that the blood-serum of affected persons so frequently has an agglutinative action upon the paratyphoid bacillus. This would not be the case if the symptoms were due to toxic substances alone. Altogether the role of toxins formed by B. enteritidis and its allies in food outside the body cannot be said to be established. The available evidence points to infection as the main, if not the sole, way in which the bacilli of this group are harmful.

Sources of infection.--The main sources of enteritidis-suipestifer infection are: (1) diseased domestic animals, the infected flesh or milk of which is used for food; (2) infection of food by human carriers during the process of preparation or serving. To these may be added a third possibility: (3) contamination of food with bacteria of this group which are inhabitants of the normal animal intestine. Considering these in order:

1. Diseased animals: The majority of the meat poisoning outbreaks are caused by meat derived from pigs or cattle. Table III gives the figures for a number of British[77] and German[78] epidemics.

TABLE III[79]

```
===============================================================
===== | | | BELONGING TO | B. ENTERITIDIS | B. SUIPESTIFER | THIS GROUP
BUT | | |UNDIFFERENTIATED |--------------------+--------------------+----------------
|British|German|Total|British|German|Total| British ---------+-------+------+----
-+-------+------+-----+---------------- Pig | 1 | 1 | 2 | 3 | 5 | 8 | 4 Ox or cow| 3 | 9
| 12 | 2 | 3 | 5 | 5 Calf | 0 | 7 | 7 | 2 | 2 | 4 | 0 Horse | 0 | 1 | 1 | 0 | 1 | 1 | ...
Chickens | 1 | 0 | 1 | 0 | 1 | 1 | ... -------------------------------------------------------------
-----------
```

Occasional outbreaks have also been attributed to infection through eating rabbit, sheep, goose, fish, shrimp, and oysters. Especially noteworthy is the relative rarity of infection from the meat of the sheep.

More definite information is needed respecting the pathological conditions caused by these bacteria in animals and the relation of such conditions to subsequent human infection. A rather remarkable problem is presented by the relation of B. suipestifer to hog cholera. This bacillus, although not now considered the causal agent of hog cholera, is very commonly associated with the disease as an accessory or secondary invader, and is frequently found in the internal organs of swine after death. It might be supposed that in regions where hog cholera is prevalent human infections would be more common than in other districts, but this seems not to be the case. No connection has ever been demonstrated between outbreaks of hog cholera--in which B. suipestifer is known to be abundantly distributed--and so-called B. suipestifer infections in man.

Suppurative processes in cattle, and especially in calves, have given rise to poisoning from the use of the meat or milk of the infected animals. It has been often demonstrated that bacteria of the enteritidis-suipestifer group are associated with inflammation of the udder in cows and with a variety of septicemic conditions in cattle and other domestic animals as well as with manifestations of intestinal disturbances ("calf diarrhea," etc.).[80] The frequency with which poisoning has occurred through the use of the meat of "emergency-slaughtered" animals has been already mentioned. K. F. Meyer[81] has reported an instance of accidental infection in a laboratory worker caused by handling a bottle of sterilized milk that had been artificially contaminated with a pure culture of B. enteritidis for experimental purposes. The strain responsible for the infection had been isolated from the heart blood of a calf that had succumbed to infectious diarrhea.

2. Human contamination: In a certain number of paratyphoid food infections there is some evidence that the food was originally derived from a healthy animal and became infected from human sources during the process of preparation. In addition to the instances already mentioned (Reinhold et al., p. 67) the Wareham (England, 1910) epidemic[82] was considered by the investigators to be due to infection of meat pies by a cook who was later proved to be a carrier of paratyphoid bacilli. The evidence in this case, however, is not altogether conclusive. S鰀erbaum[83] mentions a milk-borne paratyphoid epidemic occurring in Kristiania which was ascribed to infection of the milk by a woman milker. Sacqu 間閑 and Bellot[84] report an interesting paratyphoid outbreak involving nineteen out of two hundred and fifty men in a military corps. The patients fell ill on different dates between June 14 and June 21.

It was found that an assistant cook who had been in the kitchen for several months had been attacked a little before the epidemic explosion by some slight malady which was not definitely diagnosed. He had been admitted to the hospital and was discharged convalescent. The cook, on being recalled and quarantined, stated that some days before June 10 he was indisposed with headache and anorexia. He had nevertheless continued his service in the kitchen.... B. paratyphosus B (B. suipestifer) was repeatedly found in his stools in August, September, and October.... In all probability, therefore, the outbreak was due to food contaminated by a paratyphoid-carrier who had passed through an abortive attack of the fever.[85]

Bainbridge and Dudfield[86] describe an outbreak of acute gastro-enteritis occurring in a boarding-house; it was found that no one article of food had been eaten by all the persons affected, and there were other reasons for supposing the outbreak to be due to miscellaneous food contamination by a servant who was a carrier.

There is, therefore, ground for believing that occasional contamination of food may be brought about by bacteria of this group derived from human sources. It is not clear, however, how frequent this source of infection is, compared to infection originating in diseased animals. It must be admitted, too, that English investigators are disposed to look upon outbreaks similar to those just described as infections with B. paratyphosus B, an organism which they would distinguish from the "true" food poisoning bacilli, B. enteritidis and B. suipestifer.

3. Miscellaneous contaminations: Some investigators, especially certain German writers, regard the bacilli of the paratyphoid group as so widely distributed in nature that any attempt to control the spread of infection is like fighting windmills. According to this view the bacilli occur commonly in our everyday surroundings and thence make their way rather frequently into a variety of foodstuffs. Various German investigators have reported the presence of paratyphoid bacilli in the intestinal contents of apparently normal swine, cattle, rats, and mice and more rarely of other animals, in water and ice, in German sausage and chopped meat, and in the bodies of apparently healthy men. To what extent their alleged ubiquity is due to

mistaken bacterial identification, as claimed by some English investigators, remains to be proved. There is no doubt that in some quarters exaggerated notions have prevailed respecting a wide distribution of the true paratyphoid bacteria. Savage and others believe that the hypothesis that food poisoning outbreaks are derived from ordinary fecal infection of food is quite unfounded. It is pointed out that there is good evidence of the frequent occurrence of intestinal bacteria in such food as sausages and chopped meat, and that consequently, if paratyphoid infections could occur through ordinary contamination with intestinal bacteria not connected with any specific animal infection, food poisoning outbreaks should be exceedingly common instead of--as is the case--comparatively rare.

At the present time even those who maintain that these bacilli are of common occurrence admit that their abundance is more marked in some regions than in others. Southwest Germany, for example, seems to harbor paratyphoid bacilli in relatively large numbers. Possibly local differences in distribution may account for the discrepancies in the published findings of German and British investigators.

A special case is presented by the relation of these bacilli to rats and mice. Among the large number of bacteria of the paratyphoid group is the so-called Danysz bacillus, an organism quite pathogenic for rodents, and now and again used in various forms as a "rat virus" for purposes of rodent extermination. Several outbreaks of food poisoning in man have been attributed on more or less cogent evidence to food contamination by one of these viruses either directly by accident, as in the case described by Shibayama,[87] in which cakes prepared for rats were eaten by men, or indirectly through food contaminated by mice or rats that had been infected with the virus.[88] The use of such viruses has not proved of very great practical value in the destruction of rodents, and is open to serious sanitary objections, since the animals after apparent recovery can continue to carry the bacilli of the virus and to distribute them on or near food substances.

It seems possible that rats and mice may become infected with certain bacteria of this group without human intervention, and that these infected animals may be the means of contaminating foodstuffs and so causing outbreaks of food poisoning. Proof of the frequency with which this actually occurs is naturally difficult to obtain.

There is no escape from the conclusion that in any given case of food poisoning the exact source of infection is often largely conjectural. Even when suspicion falls strongly on a particular article of food, it may not be possible to establish beyond a reasonable doubt whether the material (meat or milk) came from a diseased animal or whether it was infected from other sources (man or other animals) at some stage during the process of preparation and serving. The most definitely attested cases yet put on record are those in which it is possible to trace the infection to food derived from an ailing animal.

Means of prevention.--The most obvious and probably the most important method of preventing infection with paratyphoid bacilli is the adoption of a system of inspection which will exclude from the market as far as possible material from infected animals. To be most effective such inspection must be directed to examination of the living animal. The milk or the meat from diseased animals may give no visible sign of abnormality. In the Ghent outbreak of 1895 the slaughter-house inspector, a veterinary surgeon, was so firmly convinced that the meat which he had passed could have had no connection with the outbreak, that he ate several pieces to demonstrate its wholesomeness. The experiment had a tragic ending, as the inspector was shortly attacked with severe choleraic symptoms and died five days later, paratyphoid bacilli being found at the autopsy. M 鼺 ler[89] also has described a case in which paratyphoid bacilli were found in meat that had given rise to a meat poisoning outbreak although the meat was normal in appearance and the organs of the animal showed no evidence of disease to the naked eye. It is evident that inspection of the live animal will often reveal evidence of disease which might be missed in the ordinary examination of slaughter-house products.

Although inspection of cows used for milking and of food animals before slaughter is highly important, it does not constitute an absolute protection. Emphasis must be repeatedly laid on the fact that meat, and especially milk that is derived from seemingly healthy animals, may nevertheless contain paratyphoid bacilli. To meet this difficulty in part the direct bacterial examination of the carcasses of slaughtered food animals has been proposed, but this seems hardly practicable as a general measure. In spite of all precautions taken at the time of slaughtering it seems probable that occasionally paratyphoid-infected meat will pass the first line of defense and be placed on the market.

This danger, which is probably not a very grave one under a reasonably good system of inspection of live animals, may be met by thoroughly cooking all foods of animal origin. It is worth noting that some of the internal organs, as the liver and kidneys, are more likely to contain bacteria than the masses of muscle commonly eaten as "meat." Sausages, from their composition and mode of preparation, and chopped meat ("hamburger steak") are also to be treated with especial care. Consumption of such foods as raw sausage or diseased goose liver (pat?de foie gras) involves a relatively high risk. It is true of paratyphoid infection as of most other forms of food poisoning that thorough cooking of food greatly diminishes the likelihood of trouble.

Whatever be the precise degree of danger from food infection by healthy paratyphoid-carriers (man or domestic animals), it is obvious that general measures of care and cleanliness will be more or less of a safeguard. As with typhoid fever so all outbreaks of paratyphoid should be thoroughly investigated in order that the sources of infection may be found and eliminated. The possible connection of rats and mice with these outbreaks should furnish an additional incentive to lessen the number of such vermin as well as to adopt measures of protecting food against their visits.

FOOTNOTES:

[62] Fleischvergiftungen u. Paratyphusinfektionen (Jena, 1910).

[63] Rept. to Local Govt. Board, N.S. No. 77 (London, 1913).

[64] Zeit. f. Hyg., XXII (1896), 53.

[65] Brit. Med. Jour., I (1909), 1171.

[66] Bernstein and Fish, Jour. Amer. Med. Assoc., LXVI (1916), 167.

[67] Breslau aerztl. Ztschr., X (1888), 249.

[68] Bernstein and Fish, Jour. Amer. Med. Assoc., LXVI (1916), 167.

[69] Deutsche Viertelj. fentl. Ges., XLV (1913), 58-59.

[70] Op. cit., pp. 60-62.

[71] Jour. Infect. Dis., XX (1917), 457.

[72] Centralbl. f. Bakt., I Orig., LIII (1910), 377.

[73] Cor.-Bl. f. schweiz. Aerzte, XLII (1912), 281 and 332.

[74] Jour. Hyg., XII (1912), 1.

[75] See Sobernheim and Seligmann, Centralbl. f. Bakt., Ref., Beilage, L (1911), 134.

[76] Report Med. Officer of Health (Newcastle-upon-Tyne, 1913).

[77] Compiled from Savage, Report of Local Gov't Board, 1913.

[78] Mayer, Deutsche Viertelj. fentl. Ges., XLV (1913), 8.

[79] It must be noted that origin of the food from a diseased animal was not definitely proved in all the cases cited. Some of these cases should possibly be classed under human contamination (2).

[80] Although not directly connected with the question of food poisoning, it is of interest to note that certain diseases of birds have been traced to infection with members of this group of bacteria. In a few cases, as in several epidemics among parrots in Paris and elsewhere, the infection has been communicated to man by contact.

[81] Jour. Infect. Dis., XIX (1916), 700.

[82] R. Trommsdorff, L. Rajchman, and A. E. Porter, Jour. Hyg., XI (1911), 89.

[83] Hygiea, LXXV (1913), 1.

[84] Program, 3d series, XXVI (1910), 25.

[85] Ledingham and Arkwright, The Carrier Problem in Infectious Diseases, pp. 152-53.

[86] Jour. Hyg., XI (1911), 24.

[87] Munch. med. Wchnschr., LIV (1907), 979.

[88] See, for example, H. Langer and Thomann, Deutsche med. Wchnschr., XL (1914), 493.

[89] Ztschr. f. Infektionsk. ... d. Haustiere, VIII (1910), 237.

CHAPTER VII

ANIMAL PARASITES

Not only pathogenic bacteria but certain kinds of animal parasites sometimes enter the human body in or upon articles of food. One of the most important of these is the parasite causing trichiniasis.

TRICHINIASIS

Trichiniasis or trichinosis is a disease characterized by fever, muscular pains, an enormous increase in the eosinophil blood corpuscles, and other more or less well-defined symptoms; at the onset it is sometimes mistaken by physicians for typhoid fever. The responsible parasite is a roundworm (Trichinella spiralis, formerly known as Trichina) which is swallowed while in its encysted larval stage in raw or imperfectly cooked pork.[90] The cysts or envelopes in which the parasites live are dissolved by the digestive fluids and the young larvae which are liberated develop in the small intestine to the adult worm, usually within two days. The young embryos, which are produced in great numbers by the mature worms, gain entrance to the lymph channels and blood stream, and after about ten days begin to invade the muscles--a procedure which gives rise to many of the most characteristic symptoms of the infection. It is estimated that in severe cases as many as fifty million embryos may enter the circulation. The parasites finally quiet down and become encysted in the muscle tissue and the symptoms, as a rule, gradually subside. Ingestion of a large number of parasites at one time often results fatally, the mortality from trichiniasis being on the average somewhat over 5 per cent and rising in some outbreaks to a much higher figure (30 per cent). On the other hand, many infections are so light as to pass unnoticed. Williams[91] found Trichinella embryos present in 5.4 per cent of the bodies of persons dying from other causes. Such findings are considered to indicate that occasional slight Trichinella infections even in the United States are quite common. This might indeed be expected from the frequent occurrence of infection in swine, about 6 per cent of these animals being found to harbor the parasite.

[Illustration: FIG. 7.--Trichinae encysted in intercostal muscle of pig. (About 35?.) (After Neumann and Mayer.)]

The specific symptoms (such as the muscular pain) of trichiniasis may be due in part to mechanical damage of the muscle tissue, but it is also probable that they are partly due to toxic products exuded by the worms and partly to the introduction of alien protein material--the protein of the worm--into the tissues. Secondary bacterial infection is also a possibility, but there is little evidence to prove that this is an important factor in most cases of trichiniasis. The various stages observed in the progress of the disease are plainly connected with the different phases of the worm's development--the initial localization in the intestines, the invasion of the muscles, and the final encystment.

Swine become infected with this parasite by eating scraps of infected meat, or the offal of their own kind, or by eating infected rats. The rat, through its cannibalistic propensities, becomes infected frequently, and is one of the chief factors in the wide dissemination of the disease. Human infection is practically accidental and self-limited; biologically speaking, man as a host does not enter into the calculations of the parasite.

Treatment of established trichiniasis infection is palliative, not truly remedial. The parasites, once inside the body, cannot be materially affected by the administration of any drug. While cure of trichiniasis is thus difficult, if not impossible, prevention is very simple. The thorough cooking of all food is sufficient to preclude infection. This relatively simple means of destroying the larvae is a more certain as well as less expensive method of preventing infection than is the laborious microscopic examination of the tissues of every slaughtered hog. In Germany between 1881 and 1898 over 32 per cent of 6,329 cases of trichinosis that were investigated were traced to meat that had been microscopically examined and passed as free from trichinae.[92] On the other hand, thorough cooking removes all possibility of danger.

TENIASIS

Various tapeworm or cestode infections are contracted by eating meat containing the parasite. Particular species of tapeworm usually infest the flesh of specific hosts, as Tenia saginata in the beef and Tenia solium in the hog. The dwarf tapeworm, Hymenolepis nana, develops in rats, and the human infections with this parasite occasionally observed are probably caused by contamination of food by these animals.

[Illustration: FIG. 8.--Cysticercus cellulosae in pig's tongue. (After Neumann and Mayer.)]

Sometimes the existence of the tapeworm in man is restricted to the alimentary tract and the symptoms vary from trivial to severe, but sometimes (Tenia solium) the larval stage of the tapeworm invades the tissues and becomes encysted in various organs (brain, eye, etc.), where, as in the case of cerebral infection, it may result fatally. The encysted larva of Tenia solium was at one time regarded as an independent animal species and named Cysticercus cellulosae. The condition known as "measly pork" is produced by the occurrence of this encysted parasite.

So-called hydatid disease is due to the cystic growth produced by the larva of a species of tapeworm (Echinococcus) inhabiting the intestine of the dog. Human infection may be caused by contaminated food as well as more directly by hands soiled with petting infected dogs. Several varieties of tapeworms infesting fish, especially certain fresh-water species, may be introduced into the human body in raw or partly cooked fish.

Methods for the prevention of tapeworm infection include the destruction of the larvae by heat--that is, the thorough cooking of all meat and fish--and the minimization of close contact with those animals, such as the dog and cat, that are likely to harbor parasites. Cleanliness in the preparation and serving of food, and attention to hand-washing before meals, and especially after touching pet animals, are necessary corollaries.

UNCINARIASIS

Hookworm infection (uncinariasis, ankylostomiasis) is commonly caused by infection through the skin of the feet, but the possibility of mouth infection cannot be disregarded, and in regions where hookworm disease exists methods of guarding against food contamination should be practiced, as well as other precautions. Billings and Hickey[93] believe that hookworm disease is contracted by unconscious coprophagy (from raw vegetables) much more frequently than is generally supposed.

OTHER PARASITES

A number of other parasitic worms (e.g., Strongyloides, Ascaris or eelworm, and Oxyuria or pinworm) may conceivably enter the human body in contaminated food, and while, as in hookworm disease, other modes of infection are probably more important, the liability to occasional infection by uncooked food must not be overlooked.

[Illustration: FIG. 9.--Lamblia intestinalis. (After Neumann and Mayer.)]

Various forms of dysentery or diarrhea have been attributed to infection with Giardia (Lamblia) intestinalis. Observations made by Fantham and Porter[94] upon cases contracted in Gallipoli and Flanders have given support to this view. Strains of this parasite of human origin have been shown to be pathogenic for mice and kittens. It is considered possible that these animals may act as reservoirs of infection and spread the disease by contamination of human food.

FOOTNOTES:

[90] The consumption of raw sausage made with pig meat is particularly likely to give rise to trichiniasis.

[91] Jour. Med. Research, VI (1901), 64.

[92] Edelmann, Mohler, and Eichhorn, Meat Hygiene, 1916, p. 182.

[93] Jour. Amer. Med. Assoc., LXVII (1916), 1908.

[94] Brit. Med. Jour., II (1916), 139.

CHAPTER VIII

POISONOUS PRODUCTS FORMED IN FOOD BY BACTERIA AND OTHER MICRO-ORGANISMS

In close relation to the cases of infection with animal or plant parasites which have been discussed, there are certain well-established instances of poisoning by substances that have been generated in food while it is still outside of the body. This is the common type of food poisoning in popular estimation, but in point of fact the proved cases of this class are much less frequent than the instances of true infection with bacteria of the paratyphoid-enteritidis group (chapter vi). Thus far the best-known examples of poisoning by the products of micro-organisms are botulism and ergotism.

ERGOTISM

Ergotism or ergot poisoning is due to the use of rye that has become diseased through the attack of a fungus, Claviceps purpurea. It occurred frequently in the Middle Ages when in times of famine the ergot or spurred rye (O.Fr. argot, "a cock's spur") was often used in default of better food. In Limoges in 922 it is said that forty thousand persons perished from this cause. Improvement in the facilities for transportation of food into regions where crops have failed, and the use of special methods for separating the diseased grain from the wholesome have greatly reduced the prevalence of ergotism. In Western Europe poisoning from this cause has practically ceased, although Hirsch recorded some twenty-eight outbreaks in the nineteenth century; in parts of Russia the disease is said still to occur in years of bad harvest.[95]

The poison ergot itself has long been used as a drug in obstetrics, but its composition is complex and is still not completely understood. Several constituents of ergot have been extracted, and these have been shown to possess different physiological effects.[96] The symptoms observed in the outbreaks of ergotism of mediaeval times are not wholly reproduced experimentally by the drug and are thought to have been in part due to the semi-starvation engendered by the use of rye from which the nutritious portions had been largely removed by the growth of the fungus.

BOTULISM

The best established case of poisoning by means of bacterial products taken in with the food is the serious malady known somewhat inappropriately as botulism (botulus, sausage).[97] This kind of food poisoning, which has a characteristic set of symptoms, seems to have been first recognized and described in 1820 by the German poet and medical writer Justinus Kerner. In two articles (1820-22) he enumerates 174 cases with 71 deaths occurring in W 黯 ttemberg between 1793 and 1822 and apparently in most cases connected with the use of insufficiently smoked sausage. Mayer[98] tabulates about 600 additional cases observed in various parts of Germany down to the end of 1908, the total mortality in the 800 cases being about 25 per cent. In France botulism is said to be very rare.[99] In Great Britain Savage[100] declares that he has been unable to trace the occurrence of a single outbreak. In the United States several instances of botulism poisoning are on record (Sheppard,[101] 1907, 3 cases, 3 deaths, canned pork and beans; Peck,[102] 1910, 12 cases, 11 deaths; Wilbur and Orpheus,[103] 1914, canned string beans, 12 cases, 1 death; Frost,[104] 1915, 3 cases, 3 deaths). Professor Stiles[105] has given a graphic description of his own attack of probable botulism due in all likelihood to minced chicken.

Symptoms.--The description of a case seen by Wilbur and Orpheus,[106] is so typical that it may be cited:

Girl, aged 23, Tuesday evening, Nov. 23, 1913, ate the dinner including the canned string beans of the light green color together with a little rare roast beef. The following day she felt perfectly normal except that at 10:00 in the evening the eyes felt strained after some sewing. Thursday morning, thirty-six hours after the meal, when the patient awoke, the eyes were out of focus, appetite was not good, and she felt very tired. At night she had still no appetite, was nauseated, and vomited the noon meal apparently undigested. Friday morning, two and one-half days after the meal, the eyes were worse, objects being seen double on quick movement, and it was noticed that they had a tendency to be crossed. A peculiar mistiness of vision was also complained of. She was in bed until late in the afternoon, when she visited Dr. Black. She had had some disturbance in swallowing previous to this time and stated that it felt as if "something came up from below" that interfered with deglutition. The fourth day she remained in bed, was much constipated, and noticed a marked decrease in the amount of urine voided. There was at no time pain except for occasional mild abdominal cramps, no headache, subnormal temperature, and a normal pulse. The fourth and fifth days the breathing became difficult at times and swallowing was almost impossible. The patient complained of a dry throat with annoying thirst. The sixth day there were periods of a sense of suffocation with a vague feeling of unrest and as if there might be difficulty in getting the next breath. The upper lids had begun to droop. The voice was nasal. When the attempt was made to swallow liquids they passed back through the nose. The patient felt markedly weak.

Physical examination at this time showed ptosis of both upper eyelids, dilatation of the right pupil, sluggish reaction to light of both pupils, apparent paralysis of the internal rectus of the left eye, normal retina, inability to raise the head, control apparently having been lost of the muscles of the neck, inability to swallow, absence of taste. The tongue was heavily coated and the throat was covered with a viscid whitish mucus clinging to the mucous membrane. The soft palate could be raised but was sluggish, particularly on the right side. The exudate on the right tonsil was so marked that it resembled somewhat a diphtheritic membrane. The seventh day there was some change in the condition; occasional periods occurred when swallowing was more effective, and there was less tendency to strangle. On the eleventh day there was some improvement of the eyes, still strangling on swallowing, sensation of taste was keener, and the general condition improved. The twelfth day the patient was able to move her head, but was unable to lift it except when she took hold of the braids of her hair, and pulled the head forward. The eyes could be opened slightly, speech was less nasal and more distinct, and improvement in swallowing was marked. At the end of two weeks the patient was able to take soft diet freely, and at four weeks she was up in a chair for a couple of hours complaining only of general weakness and inability to use her eyes. At the end of five weeks she was able to leave the hospital and return to her home and later to resume her regular work.

In all cases the nervous system is strikingly affected in this form of food poisoning. Dizziness, double vision, difficulty in chewing and swallowing, and other symptoms of nervous involvement occur with varying intensity and may persist for a long time after the first signs of the attack. Temperature, pulse, and respiration remain practically normal. In contrast with the traditional type of food poisoning gastro-intestinal symptoms may be slight or altogether lacking. Freedom from abdominal pain is usually noted; diarrhea is the exception and constipation the rule; vomiting sometimes occurs, but may be absent. In the cases described by Sheppard there was "an entire absence of the usual gastro-intestinal symptoms from first to last, no pain or sensory disturbance and no elevation of temperature." The visual disturbances are very characteristic. Stiles relates his own experiences as follows:

Vertigo and nystagmus developed [a few hours after eating] in a startling degree, the car [in which he was being taken to his house] seemed to be ascending an endless spiral, the stars made circles in the sky, and the houses by the wayside reeled. The lighted doorway of my house seemed to approach and surround me as I was carried in. My bed for the moment presented itself as a vertical surface which I could not conceive to be a resting place.... Whenever I opened my eyes on this day [the next day] the impression of gyration of the room was appalling.... To turn my head even very slowly from one side to the other brought an accession of the overpowering giddiness.... [eight days after the beginning of the attack]. The nystagmus now became limited to momentary onsets, but in its place I became aware of a peculiar diplopia. The image of one retina was not merely displaced from the position of its fellow but was tilted about 15 degrees from parallel.... This fantastic diplopia gradually gave place to the familiar variety and this occurred less and less often as my convalescence proceeded. From [this date] my recovery pursued a course which was dishearteningly slow but free from any setbacks. Among the persistent symptoms were ... the visual difficulties mentioned. The left pupil was usually smaller than the right and I thought I detected a slight failure to relax accommodation with the left eye. Reading was difficult for several weeks and the ability to write, as requiring closer fixation, was still longer in returning.

In the cases reported by Sheppard visual symptoms were the initial signs of trouble, double vision, mistiness, and inability to hit the mark in shooting being the first complaint.

The time elapsing between eating the implicated food and the onset of the earliest symptoms is usually between twelve and forty-eight hours, but may be much less. In Stiles's case the interval was apparently less than three hours.

Anatomical lesions.--In fatal cases no characteristic gross changes are observed in the various organs. It has been stated by some writers that microscopic degenerative changes occur in the ganglion cells, involving especially the so-called Nissl granules, but in the carefully studied case reported by Orpheus[107] the Nissl granules were quite normal in size, arrangement, and staining qualities. There was, in fact, no evidence to substantiate the hypothesis of a specific action of the toxin on the nerve-cells. On the other hand, Orpheus found numerous hemorrhages in the brain-stem and multiple thromboses in both the arteries and veins. He holds, consequently, that the indications of severe disturbances of brain circulation associated with hemorrhages and thrombosis in medulla and pons are sufficient to explain the symptoms of botulism poisoning without having recourse to the assumption that the poison has a specific action on certain ganglion cells.

Bacteriology.--The cause of botulism poisoning was discovered by Van Ermengem to be the toxin produced by a bacillus which he named B. botulinus. This organism was isolated from portions of a ham that had caused fifty cases of poisoning (1895) at Ellezelles (Belgium), and also from the spleen and gastric contents of one of the three fatal cases. The bacillus grows only in the absence of oxygen (strict anaerobe), stains by Gram's method, forms terminal spores, and develops best at 22. Unlike most bacteria dangerous to man, it appears unable to grow in the human body, and its injurious effect is limited to the action of the toxin produced in foodstuffs outside the body. Botulism is an intoxication--not an infection. The fact that the bacillus can grow in nature only when the free oxygen supply is cut off explains in part at least the relatively rare occurrence of botulism since all the conditions necessary for the production of the botulism toxin do not commonly concur. Next to nothing is known as to how widely B. botulinus is distributed. Except in connection with the cases of poisoning it has been reported but once in nature.[108] The botulism poison is a true bacterial toxin, chemically unstable, destroyed by heating at 80. for 30 minutes, capable of provoking violent symptoms in minute doses, and possessing the property characteristic of all true toxins of generating an antitoxin when injected in small, non-fatal doses into the bodies of susceptible animals. In animal experiments the toxin formed by B. botulinus has been found capable of reproducing the typical clinical picture of this form of food poisoning. Symptoms of paralysis are produced in rabbits, guinea-pigs, and other animals by the injection of so small a dose as 0.0001 c.c. of a filtered broth culture.

Epidemiology.--The conditions under which B. botulinus occurs and is given opportunities for multiplying are not completely known. It is possible that there are localities where this bacillus is particularly abundant in the soil or in the intestinal contents of swine or other domestic animals, but on the whole it seems more probable that the organism is widely distributed, but that it does not often find suitable conditions for entrance into, and multiplication in, human food. Practically all the reported cases of botulism have been caused by food which has been given some sort of preliminary treatment, as smoking, pickling, or canning, then allowed to stand for a time, and eaten before cooking. Since both the bacillus, including the spore stage, and its toxin are destroyed by relatively slight heating, it is clear that a rather unusual set of factors must co-operate in order that botulism poisoning shall take place. These are evidently: (1) the presence of the bacilli in sufficient numbers in a suitable foodstuff; (2) the initial preparation of the food by a method that does not destroy the B. botulinus--inadequate smoking, too weak brine,[109] or insufficient cooking; (3) the holding of this inadequately preserved food for a sufficient length of time under the right conditions of temperature and lack of oxygen; (4) the use of this food, in which conditions have conspired to favor the production of toxin by B. botulinus, without final adequate cooking. It seems as reasonable to suppose that the infrequency with which these several factors coincide is responsible for the relative uncommonness of botulism as to suppose it due to the rarity of the specific bacillus. In the Belgian outbreak studied by Van Ermengem the poisonous ham had lain at the bottom of a cask of brine (anaerobic conditions) while the other ham of the same animal lay on top of it but was not covered with brine, and was eaten without producing any poisonous effect. In this instance the presence or absence of favorable conditions for anaerobic growth seemed to be the decisive factor.

Prevention and treatment.--The food in which B. botulinus has grown does not seem to be altered in a way that necessarily arouses suspicion. In the case described, the incriminated ham showed bluish-gray areas from which B. botulinus could be isolated, but this condition does not seem to have attracted attention before the poisoning occurred and was an observation made only after the event. So far as can be learned the meat that has caused botulism has always come from perfectly sound animals. In some cases the accused article of food is said to have had a rancid or acrid taste (due to butyric acid?), but there is nothing definitely characteristic about this, as the majority of anaerobes produce butyric acid. If, as in the Darmstadt[110] and Stanford University[111] epidemics, the food (canned beans) is served with salad dressing, a sour taste might pass without notice or even add to the relish. In the instance reported by Sheppard the canned beans were good in appearance, taste, and smell.

The obvious precaution to take against poisoning of this sort is first the use of adequate methods of food preservation. To judge from the recorded outbreaks, domestically prepared vegetables and meats are more likely to give rise to botulism than those prepared commercially on a large scale. The general use of steam under pressure in the large canning factories affords a high degree of protection against the anaerobic bacteria and their resistant spores. Whatever the method of treatment, all canned or preserved food having an unnatural appearance, taste, or odor should be rejected. Reheating of all prepared foods immediately before use is an additional safeguard. Foods, such as salads, composed wholly or in part of uncooked materials should not be allowed to stand overnight before being served.

If symptoms of botulism, such as visual disturbances, become manifest, the stomach should be emptied with a stomach pump, cathartics administered, and strychnine and other stimulants given as required. Since one of the noteworthy features of this disease is the paralysis of the intestinal tract by the toxin absorbed, the guilty food may lie for a long time in the stomach (cf. Stiles, loc. cit.). Consequently, measures to empty the stomach should be taken even if the patient does not come under observation until several days after the poisonous food has been eaten.

An antitoxic serum has been prepared at the Koch Institute in Berlin. This serum has given successful results in animal experimentation, but has not been used, so far as I can learn, in any human outbreak. It is not available at any point in this country.

OTHER BACTERIAL POISONS

The interesting case reported by Barber[112] shows that there are other possibilities of food poisoning by formed bacterial poisons. Acute attacks of gastro-enteritis were produced in several individuals by the use of milk containing a poisonous substance elaborated by a white staphylococcus. This staphylococcus occurred in almost pure culture in the udder of the cow from which the milk was derived. The milk when used fresh was harmless and the poison was generated in effective quantities only when the milk stood some hours at room temperature before being used. The symptoms were similar to those usually ascribed to "ptomain poisoning."

SPOILED AND DECOMPOSED FOOD

There is a general belief that food is unwholesome whenever the evidence of the senses shows it to be more or less decomposed. This opinion finds expression in civilized countries in many legal enactments forbidding traffic in decomposed meats, vegetables, and fruits. There is unfortunately lack of evidence as to what kinds or degree of visible decomposition are most dangerous. In fact, some foods of high nutrient value, notably cheeses, are eaten only after somewhat extensive decomposition processes (termed ripening) have taken place. The characteristic flavors or aromas of the various hard and soft cheeses are due to the substances formed by certain species of molds and bacteria and are just as properly to be regarded as decomposition products as the unpleasant stenches generated by decomposing eggs or meat. Indeed, some of the decomposition products formed in the ripening of Brie, Camembert, or Limburger are similar to, if not identical with, those which are associated with spoiled foods. Sour milk, again, is recommended and commonly used as a food or beverage for persons in delicate health, and yet sour milk contains many millions of bacteria and their decomposition products. Some of the bacteria commonly concerned in the natural souring of milk are closely related to pathogenic types. The partial decomposition of meats and game birds is often considered to be advantageous rather than otherwise. Even eggs, a food whose "freshness" is marred for most persons by the initial stages of decomposition, are ripened in various ways by the Chinese and eaten as a delicacy after the lapse of months or years. The preserved ducks' eggs known as pidan are stored for months in a pasty mixture of tea, lime, salt, and wood ashes. "They are very different from fresh eggs. The somewhat darkened shell has numerous dark green dots on the inner membrane. Both the white and yolk are coagulated; the white is brown, more or less like coffee jelly...."[113] Increase of ammoniacal nitrogen has taken place to an extraordinary degree in these eggs, indicating much decomposition of the egg protein. The ammoniacal nitrogen in pidan is considerably higher than in the eggs known by egg candlers as black rots.

It is evident, therefore, that bacterial growth in substances used as food is not necessarily injurious and may in some cases increase the palatability of food without destroying its wholesomeness. Little or nothing is known about the correlation of visible signs of decomposition with the presence of poisonous products, and it is at present impossible to say at what point in the process of decomposition a food becomes unfit to use owing to the accumulation of poisonous substances within it. There seems to be no connection between the natural repugnance to the use of a food and its unwholesomeness. Under ordinary conditions the nauseous character of very stale eggs is proverbial, and yet few nitrogenous foods have so clear a health record as eggs or have been so infrequently connected with food poisoning outbreaks.

It might seem tempting to conclude on the basis of the available evidence that spoiled or decomposed foods possess poisonous qualities only when certain specific bacteria, like the B. botulinus already discussed, have accidentally invaded them and formed definite and specific poisons. But we have no right to assume that the everyday decomposition products of the banal bacteria are in all cases without injurious effects. Even though no sharply defined acute form of poisoning may be laid at their door, it does not follow that an irritating or perhaps slightly toxic action of the ordinary decomposition products is altogether absent. Our present knowledge of the nature and degree of danger to be apprehended from the use of spoiled food is imperfect and unsatisfactory. That fact, however, does not release us from the obligation to continue measures of protection based even to a limited extent on experience.

FOOTNOTES:

[95] Another species of Claviceps (C. paspali) which attacks the seeds of a wild grass is believed to be responsible for certain outbreaks of poisoning among cattle and horses (Science, XLIII [1916], 894).

[96] Barger (Jour. Chem. Soc., XCV [1909], 1123) has shown that parahydroxyphenylethylamine is present in ergot and is in some degree responsible for the physiological action of the drug.

[97] Although some of the early outbreaks were traced to the use of sausage, particularly in W 鱠 ttemberg, the proportion of recent botulism poisoning attributed to this food is no greater than of sausage-conveyed infections with the paratyphoid bacillus (chap. vi), and a number of the most completely studied outbreaks of botulism have been traced to ham, beans, and other foods.

[98] Deutsche Viertelj. fentl. Ges., XLV (1913), 8.

[99] Program , XXVI (1910), 583.

[100] Report to Local Govt. Board on Bacterial Food Poisoning and Food Inspection, N.S. No. 77, 1913, p. 27.

[101] Southern Cal. Pract., XXII (1907), 370.

[102] Ibid., XXV (1910), 121.

[103] Arch. of Int. Med., XIV (1914), 589.

[104] Amer. Med., X (1915), 85.

[105] Jour. Amer. Med. Assoc., LXI (1913), 2301.

[106] Loc. cit.

[107] Loc. cit.

[108] In the feces of a healthy pig (Kempner and Pollock, Deutsche med. Wchnschr., XXIII [1897], 505).

[109] B. botulinus does not develop in media containing over 6 per cent of salt and should not be able to grow in meat properly covered in brine made with 10 per cent of salt (Centralbl. f. Bakt., XXVII [1900], 857).

[110] G. Landmann, Hyg. Rundschau, XIV (1904), 449.

[111] Wilbur and Orpheus, Arch. of Int. Med., XIV (1914), 589.

[112] Phil. Jour. of Science, IX (1914), B6, p. 515.

[113] K. Blunt and C. C. Wang, Jour. Biol. Chem., XXVIII (1916), 125.

CHAPTER IX

POISONING OF OBSCURE OR UNKNOWN NATURE

While many and diverse causes of food poisoning have been discussed in the foregoing pages, there remain certain affections definitely connected with food that are still of obscure or doubtful causation.

MILKSICKNESS OR TREMBLES

This disease, common to man and some of the higher animals, is characterized by a definite symptom-complex, the salient features being excessive vomiting and obstinate constipation accompanied usually by a subnormal temperature. Many cases result fatally. At the present time it is known to occur only rarely in some of the southern and central western states in this country, but during the period of pioneer settlement it was quite common in districts that are now seldom affected. A great many references to milksickness are found in the writings of the early travelers and physicians in the Middle West, one observer predicting that "some of the fairest portions of the West in consequence of the prevalence of this loathsome disease must ever remain an uninhabitable waste unless the cause and remedy can be discovered." In certain regions it is estimated that "nearly one-fourth of the pioneers and early settlers died of this disease." The mother of Abraham Lincoln fell a victim to this malady in 1818 in southern Indiana.

The disease appears to be usually contracted in the first instance by grazing cattle or sheep that have access to particular tracts of land; "milksickness" pastures are, as a rule, well known locally for their dangerous qualities. Milksickness is communicated to man through the medium of raw milk, or butter and possibly of meat. Although some of the earlier observers make the statement that the disease is self-propagating and can be passed on without limit from one animal to another, later experiments cast doubt on this view.[114]

Many different theories have been advanced to account for the origin of the disease. The belief that mineral poisons such as arsenic or copper might be taken up by grazing animals and eliminated in the milk finds no justification either in analytical or in clinical data. Many plants, known or suspected to be poisonous, have been accused of furnishing the substance that imparts the poisonous quality to the milk of animals suffering from trembles, but there is no agreement as to the responsible species. Feeding experiments with suspected plants have in no case given unambiguous results. While some facts have been supposed to indicate that living micro-organisms are the cause of milksickness, other facts are opposed to this view, and the most recent experiments in this direction did not lead to conclusive results.[115] The true cause of milksickness is at present quite unknown.

DEFICIENCY DISEASES

Although diseased conditions due to the absence rather than the presence of certain constituents in the food are not perhaps to be properly classed as food poisoning, they may be mentioned here to illustrate the complexity of the food problem. At least one disease,--pellagra--is attributed by some observers to the presence of an injurious substance or micro-organism in the food, and by others to the absence of certain ingredients necessary to the proper maintenance of life.

Beriberi.--One of the best established instances of a disease due to a one-sided or defective diet is beriberi. This affection is prevalent among those peoples subsisting chiefly or wholly on a diet of rice prepared in a certain way. As a matter of trade convention milled white rice has long been considered superior to the unpolished grain. The process of polishing rice by machinery removes the red husk or pericarp of the grain, and a diet based almost exclusively on polished rice causes this well-marked disease--beriberi--which was for long regarded as of an infectious nature.[116] It has been shown that if the husks are restored to the polished grain and the mixture used as food the disease fails to develop. Experiments upon chickens and pigeons show that an exclusive diet of white rice causes in these animals a disease (polyneuritis of fowls) similar to beriberi, which likewise can be arrested or prevented by a change in diet. From such observations the conclusion has been drawn that in the pericarp of the rice grain there are certain substances essential to the maintenance of health and that their withdrawal from the diet leads to nutritional disturbances. The name "vitamin" has been given to these substances, but little is known about their chemical or physiological nature. In a varied diet vitamins are presumably present in a variety of foodstuffs, but if the diet is greatly restricted, some apparently trivial treatment of the food may result in their elimination. It is uncertain how many and how various the substances are that have been classed by some writers under the designation vitamin. At least two "determinants" are thought to be concerned in the nutrition of growth, a fat-soluble and a water-soluble substance.[117]

Pellagra is one of the diseases attributed to an unbalanced diet,[118] and it has been suggested that the increased use of highly milled maize and wheat flour from which vitamins are absent may be responsible for the extension of this malady in recent years. Other observers, while admitting that a faulty diet may predispose to pellagra as to tuberculosis and other diseases, do not assent to the view that it is the primary factor.[119]

Lathyrism.--The name lathyrism has been given to a disease supposed to be connected with the use of the pulse and the chick pea. Nervous symptoms are conspicuous and sometimes severe, although the affection is of a milder type than pellagra. The disease is said to be associated with the exclusive or almost exclusive use of leguminous food and with generally miserable conditions of living. It is yet uncertain whether lathyrism is a deficiency disease like beriberi and possibly pellagra, or whether it is due to a mixture of foreign and poisonous seeds with the particular legumes consumed, or whether under certain conditions the legumes themselves may contain poisonous substances generated by some unknown fungus growths.

Favism (from fava, "bean") is an acute febrile anemia with jaundice and hemoglobinuria which occurs in Italy and has been attributed to the use of beans as food or even to smelling the blossom of the bean plant.[120] A marked individual predisposition to the malady is said to exist. Although the symptoms are very severe and seem to point to an acute poisoning, no toxic substance has been isolated from the implicated beans. It has been suggested by some that bacterial infection, and by others that a fungous growth on the bean, is responsible, but no evidence has been brought forward to support either assumption.

Scurvy in some forms is undoubtedly connected with the lack of certain necessary components of a normal diet. The development of scurvy on shipboard in the absence of fresh milk, fresh vegetables, fruit juice, and the like is a fact long familiar. Guinea-pigs fed on milk, raw and heated, and on milk and grain have developed typical symptoms of scurvy.[121] On the other hand, a form of experimental scurvy has been produced in guinea-pigs and rabbits kept on an ordinary diet of green vegetables, hay, and oats by the intravenous injection of certain streptococci.[122] The relative share of diet and infection in the production of human scurvy is consequently regarded by some investigators as uncertain.

Rachitis or rickets is a pathological condition in some way connected with a protracted disturbance of digestion which in turn leads to faulty calcium metabolism. It does not seem probable that rickets is caused by too little calcium in the food, but rather by the inability of the bone tissue to utilize the calcium brought to it in the body fluids. Experiments upon the causation of the disease have not given uniform results, and it does not seem possible at present to place responsibility for this condition upon any particular form of diet, such as deficiency of fat or excess of carbohydrates or protein. It appears to be true that the prolonged use of any food leading to nutritional disturbance causes an inability on the part of the bone cells to take up calcium salts in the normal manner.

While there are many obscure points with regard to the origin of both scurvy and rickets, there is no doubt that some dietary shortcoming lies at their base, and that they can be cured or altogether avoided by maintenance of suitable nutritional conditions.

THE FOODS MOST COMMONLY POISONOUS

Certain articles of food figure with special frequency in the reports of food poisoning outbreaks. It is not clear in all cases why this special liability to inflict injury exists. For an example, vanilla ice-cream and vanilla puddings have been so often implicated that some investigators have not hesitated to ascribe a poisonous quality to the vanilla itself. But there is no good evidence that this is the case, and it has been suggested that the reducing action of the vanilla favors the growth of anaerobic bacteria which produce poisonous substances, an explanation highly conjectural.

The conspicuous frequency with which the consumption of raw meat provokes food poisoning has already been set forth and in large part explained by the occasional derivation of meat from animals infected with parasites harmful to man. The even greater culpability of raw milk is due to the fact that milk is not only, like meat, sometimes obtained from an infected animal, but that it is a particularly good culture medium for bacteria, and in the process of collection or distribution may become infected through the agency of a human carrier. Foods such as ice-cream that are prepared with milk are also often connected with food poisoning. It seems probable that illness caused by ice-cream is much more commonly due to bacterial infection than to poisoning with metals or flavoring extracts. The responsibility of these latter substances is entirely problematic.

Cases of cheese poisoning, which apparently are relatively numerous, are of quite obscure causation. Whether such poisoning is due more commonly to some original contamination of the milk, or to an invasion of the cheese by pathogenic bacteria in the course of preparation, or to the formation of toxic substances by bacteria or molds during the process of ripening which the cheese undergoes, is left uncertain in the majority of cases.

Shellfish poisoning from eating oysters, mussels, or clams is unquestionably caused in some instances by sewage contamination of the water from which the bivalves are taken, and in such cases bacilli of the typhoid or paratyphoid groups are commonly concerned. It is a disputed question whether certain recorded outbreaks of mussel poisoning have been due to bacterial infection or whether sometimes healthy or diseased mussels taken from unpolluted water contain a poisonous substance. In a similar way it is uncertain whether a certain marine snail (Murex bradatus), sometimes used for food, contains under certain conditions a substance naturally poisonous for man, or whether it is poisonous only when it is infected or when toxigenic bacteria have grown in it.

Potato poisoning has been attributed in some cases to bacterial decomposition of potatoes by proteus bacilli; in other cases, to a poisonous alkaloid, solanin, said to be present in excessive amounts in diseased and in sprouting potatoes. It is noteworthy that many instances of potato poisoning have been connected with the use of potato salad which had stood for some time after being mixed, so that the possibility of infection with the paratyphoid bacillus or other pathogenic organisms cannot be excluded. That solanin is ever really responsible for potato poisoning is considered doubtful by many investigators.

These examples are sufficient to show that in a considerable proportion of cases of alleged food poisoning there is a large measure of uncertainty about the real source of trouble. Although the trend of opinion has been in the direction of an increased recognition of the share of certain bacteria, especially those of the paratyphoid group, there is an important residue of unexplained food poisoning that needs further skilled investigation. It is one of the objects of this book to point out this need and to draw attention to the numerous problems that await settlement. The first step is the regular and thorough investigation of every food poisoning outbreak.

FOOTNOTES:

[114] Jordan and Harris, Jour. Infect. Dis., VI (1909), 401.

[115] Ibid.

[116] E. B. Vedder, Jour. Amer. Med. Assoc., LXVII (1916), 1494.

[117] McCollum and Davis, Jour. Biol. Chem., XXIII (1915), 181.

[118] Goldberger, Jour. Amer. Med. Assoc., LXVI (1916), 471.

[119] MacNeal, Jour. Amer. Med. Assoc., LXVI (1916), 975; Jobling, Jour. Infect. Dis., XVIII (1916), 501.

[120] Gasbarrini, Policlinico, November 14, 1915; abstract, Jour. Amer. Med. Assoc., LXV (1915), 2264.

[121] Holst and Frich, Jour. Hyg., VII (1907), 619; Moore and Jackson, Jour. Amer. Med. Assoc., LXVII (1916), 1931.

[122] Jackson and Moody, Jour. Infect. Dis., XIX (1916), 511.

www.ingramcontent.com/pod-product-compliance
Lightning Source LLC
Chambersburg PA
CBHW070914180526
45168CB00005B/2010